My Journey With Breast Cancer and God's Miracles That Sustained Me

Depending On God Through Battle With Metastatic Bi-Lateral Breast Cancer

Cathy Suitor Riley

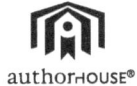

authorHOUSE®

AuthorHouse™
1663 Liberty Drive, Suite 200
Bloomington, IN 47403
www.authorhouse.com
Phone: 1-800-839-8640

First published by AuthorHouse 11/29/2007

ISBN: 978-1-4343-3170-0 (sc)

Printed in the United States of America
Bloomington, Indiana

This book is printed on acid-free paper.

ACKNOWLEDGEMENTS

-- Thank you to my husband, Bob, for being there for me when
   I was diagnosed with bi-lateral breast cancer. You will never
   know how much it meant to have you there with me. No
   one needs to be alone when they receive that devastating
   news. Thanks too for understanding when I would fall
   apart and cry. Thanks for letting me cry because that is
   just what I needed at the time. Crying cleanses our soul
   and relieves our stress, and as you know this has been a
   very stressful journey. We have been through a lot with my
   illness, but God has seen us through it. He has healed me
   and I pray that He will keep me well. I want you to always
   remember what God has done for me and should you ever
   have a critical illness I want you to remember to depend on
   God to see you through it.

-- To my special Cousins and Aunt, Lillian and Bill, Mike and
   Teretha and Aunt Lillian for all of your prayers and words
   of encouragement to me during this illness and treatment
   process.. I am truly blessed to have you for my family. Your
   prayers have kept me going and I know you will continue to
   send them up for me.

-- A special thank you to you, Lillian and Bill for the welcome
   you gave mom and I when we visited you after my mastectomy

had been completed. Boy the pink balloons and signs and angel, just more than I can name. You have both been so supportive and have encouraged me all along this journey.

-- Thank you to my special cousin, Ann, who called me and prayed for me and had others praying for me. I thank you especially for the memories of our childhood and teen years. Thank you so much for the beautiful prayer quilt your church made me during my cancer.

-- Thanks also to three special cousins on my husband's side, Cecelia, Jackie and Deidra for all you did for me throughout the past year and a half. You seem more like sisters to me than cousins. Thanks for your prayers and encouragement.

-- To my precious niece, Lori, for what you have meant to me since the day you were born. Thanks for being there for me during my illness and I'm so thankful you worked at the Cancer Center because it made it easier to come up there as much as I have had to come up there. I thank you, Charles, Bailey and Lauren for all the prayers you have sent up for me and I know you all will continue to pray for me. I love ya'll.

-- Thanks to a special friend and former co-worker, Jackie, for being there for me this whole journey. I have told you many times how much you mean to me but I could never tell you enough how much our 30 plus year friendship has meant to me and especially how much you have meant to me since my diagnosis of breast cancer.

-- To another friend, a childhood friend of mine, Sherrill, I thank you for cutting my wig for me that day when I was so upset I didn't know where to turn or where to go. You wouldn't even let me pay you for cutting the wig, but you did hold me while I cried. That and all the prayers you have said on the phone with me will always stay with me in my memories of you.

-- To my daughter's daddy, Randy and his family, I thank you for all of your prayers and your encouraging words to me throughout this ordeal. Your families mean the world to me still and I will always cherish my memories of you all. I want to say a special thank you to Letha and Tammie, who took me out to eat the day I had my medi-port put in my chest to begin my chemo therapy. I needed some "fun" that day to get my mind off of the upcoming treatments and what I was going to have to go through. You were both there for me when I needed you most. Also thanks to Phylis and Judy who have called and checked on me so much during my illness.

-- To the congregations at Hawkins Memorial United Methodist Church, Wesley Chapel United Methodist Church and Coopers Chapel Methodist Church, I appreciate all of your prayers and you allowing me to sing and witness as much as I have. You have been very tolerant of me as I was trying to serve my Lord and do what I felt He had called me to do. I love you each and every one. You would never let me give up.

-- Thanks to two special ladies at Coopers Chapel, Jewel and Peggy that had been through breast cancer prior to my diagnosis. You are both beautiful, vibrant, Christian women that gave me so much hope for a future....You are both survivors and when you are going through a journey like this you look for the success stories out there.

-- Thanks also to three other ladies that I know that had their journeys with cancer and are survivors that gave me hope also. They are Diane, Nancy and Louise. And thanks again Louise for the book you gave me that gave me hope for survival.

-- To my pastors, Rev. Pam Randall, Rev. Howard McKee, Rev. Gerald Chaney, Rev. Sephus Garrett, and Rev. Barry Skelton who have anointed me with oil, prayed for me and with me, encouraged me in the fact that "God is not through with me yet". You made me feel that my singing and my witnessing to the congregations was exactly the path God wanted me to take. You are all wonderful pastors and as I say in my book, "God knows what He is doing and He knows who to call to preach". I thank God that He brought each of you into my life. There is no doubt you are "God called".

-- A special thank you goes out to my daughter's fiancee, soon to be husband, John. I thank God for bringing you into Karen's life because you have made her so happy and she seems "so complete" with you. A mother wants nothing more than to see her children and grandchildren happy in this world. I know you love each other and I pray God will give you both a long and happy life together. Thanks for hanging in here with Karen and I as we have had to go through my critical illness. Thanks for being supportive to both of us. I love you dearly and will be glad to have you as my son-in-law.

-- Thank you to my friend, Shira. I am so thankful that I met you when I was volunteering at the hospital in Quitman and when I told you that I was looking for a church close to my home you told me about the church you attended, Coopers Chapel Methodist. You were part of God's plan to get me to that wonderful church where my music ministry began, and where I always feel the Spirit of the Lord. I have met such wonderful people in that church that have really made a difference in my life.

You are such a loving and Christian woman and you inspire me with your strength and faith as you have gone through the death of your husband, Pete, who I loved dearly also, and now as you watch your grandson, Weston battle cancer. You see how God has helped me through breast cancer and I hope that will give you the assurance you need that God will also take good care of you, Weston and all of your family.

-- Thanks to another Christian friend, Horace, who is the reason I ever began singing. Horace, I know you don't take the credit for me singing for my Lord now, but you told me that God used you as a tool to get me to sing. I am so thankful that He did use you and that you answered His urging to do that for me. May God bless you richly for that.

-- I appreciate you too, Diane, who is one of the best organists/ pianists I have ever met. You welcomed me with opened arms when I first came to Coopers Chapel and I felt close to you and Stanley from the very beginning. I really don't know what that church would do without you to provide the music. You and Jerry Dale do a great job and I love to hear you both play. I thank God now too for Mrs. Skelton, the pastor's wife because she is good to fill in for you.

-- A special new friend of mine, Mrs. Peggy Mosely, who I met when I was asked to speak to the Radiologic Society at Rush Hospital, I say a big thank you for allowing me to speak that night and to tell my story about my breast cancer. It did my heart good to have them tell me that "they will never look at their jobs the same again".

-- And now I want to thank all the medical people, Drs., radiologists, nurses, etc., that have been involved in the diagnosing and treatment of this terrible disease. Each of you mean so much to me in your own special way. Many of the medical staff I have come into contact with during this I don't even know their names, but you have been very good to me.

I want to say a special thank you to a wonderful Christian lady and Radiologist, Dr. Sandra Pupa, who was so wonderful to me at the time she had to tell me that I had breast cancer. You are truly an angel and God called. You have been so good to me all the way through this journey and I will never forget you.

Thank you also to Dr. Dwight Keady , the most wonderful Oncologist in the world. I have trusted you from the very beginning of this illness and I continue to trust you. Believe me it is a relief to know that I have such a competent and precious doctor fighting for my life. I could never thank you enough for taking such good care of me and allowing me to talk to you and ask questions that concern me. You never rush me through the visit. I thank God for you. May God give you a special star in your crown and special blessings for what you have done for me.

Thanks to the nurses that have taken care of me at the Cancer Center. Stephanie, Wendy, Rebecca and Marilyn. Ya'll are truly amazing. You are so friendly and caring yet you are so competent in what you are doing there. You treat all the patients the same and believe me it does not go unnoticed. I love you all and appreciate how you take such good care of me.

And thanks to all the staff at the Cancer Center from office staff, lab staff, nurses, x-ray staff, even housekeeping staff, you are all wonderful. Always friendly and smiling and making me feel so special by calling me "Aunt Cathy". I have enjoyed the blanket ya'll made me to keep me warm during chemo. I will cherish it always.

And, last but not least I want to thank Dr. William Billups, III, my surgeon. You are incredible. You did a wonderful job on my mastectomy. My scar is barely detectable twelve months after surgery. You and your nurse, Lisa, have meant so much to me throughout this difficult time in my life. I pray God will bless you as you perform future surgeries on your patients. We are truly blessed to have you as our surgeon.

DEDICATION

This book is written in memory of my daddy, Rev. Roy Suitor, my brothers, Richard, Jimmy and Buddy, my sister Peggy and my cousin, Joyce (Brenda), who was more like a sister to me than a cousin. I do have the peace in knowing that when God does call me home I will be reunited with you all whom I have missed so much since you went to the other side. What a great reunion that will be!

I would like to dedicate this book to the loving memory of my Dad, Reverend Roy A. Suitor (1907-1986), who was not only one of the best daddy's in the world but also one of the best pastors in the world. He was a wonderful Christian influence on me and so many others. He was a shining example, a living, breathing and walking testimony of our Lord and Savior, Jesus Christ.

This book is also dedicated in honor of my wonderful, Christian mother, Thelma Suitor, whose trials and tribulations served as lessons for me in building my faith in God. She was dedicated to my dad in his work for the Lord and has been a great encourager of me throughout the years and especially during my cancer.

This book is also dedicated to my daughter, Karen, who knows how much I love her and whose heart is full of love for God. I thank her for the talks that we have had that gave my heart peace to know that she is a "believer" like me, because I know that whatever comes her way in life she knows where her help comes from and will depend on God to be there for her as He has been for me. I thank Karen also for being so supportive of me during my breast cancer journey. About four months after I was diagnosed with breast cancer, Karen's boyfriend, John, proposed to her on her birthday. I am thankful that she and John found each other and that they both seem so happy with each other. They plan to marry May, 2007 and I pray God will richly bless their marriage for many years to come. I am so thankful that God has healed me so that I will be able to attend their wedding on the beach. Karen and I went shopping and she picked out a beautiful wedding dress. I told her daddy that he will be really proud of how pretty she is going to look in that dress. When they were first engaged I wasn't even sure if I would live another year to see their wedding. God has really blessed me so much and I am really looking forward to seeing them married. John has a son, Brian and he is about two years younger than Karen's son, Cody. They love each other so much already and have become like brothers. They will be involved in the wedding also and I know they will be so cute.

Last, but not least, this book is dedicated to my number one encourager, my grandson, Cody. He knows that the main reason for my wanting to live and beat this breast cancer is him. I have taught him about God's love and God's promises in the bible and when I tend to forget, Cody reminds me. I had read to him in the bible the verse that says God will put an utter end to this and the affliction shall not rise up a second time. If I make the comment that "if the cancer comes back", that ten year old little boy will rare back and look at me and say, "Memaw the bible says God will not let it rise up a second time". Thank God for Cody's faith. Cody and I have gone through this cancer journey hand in hand and I thank him for all of his support! Some of my happiest times and biggest laughs have been with him. I pray every single day that God will allow me to stay well and be able to live to see my only grandchild, Cody, grown and self sufficient. It does my heart good to know that Cody prays about everything and we have had many talks about God and prayer and I know that the memories of our talks will remain with both of us always. I love you dearly, Cody.

And finally, thanks to every person, friend or family or stranger, that spoke an encouraging word or prayer on my behalf. You will never know how much you all meant to me during this difficult time in my life. I know in my heart that God sent each and every one of you into my life at the exact time I needed a message to be delivered from Him through you. Thanks for listening to the promptings of God and following through on them. Always listen for God's guidance, because He does work through us to help others.

TABLE OF CONTENTS

INTRODUCTION

It is my hope that through this book I might touch someone's heart and soul and bring them a better understanding of how much our God loves us, knows what's best for us and performs miracles beyond our understanding.

God is as near as our next breath, He is the reason we have breath at all...He is involved in every part of our life. He knows what we are going through and is just waiting for us to turn our battles over to Him so that we come out on the other side winners and stronger in the Lord because of those trials.

Please remember that God will never leave you nor forsake you. He will take your hand and even though you may weaken or your faith may waiver, God will never let go of your hand. He will be there and go the distance with you always. Pray without ceasing, read your bible faithfully and trust me you will never walk alone - God will be right beside you!

May God bless each and every one of you as you read and meditate on this book. I pray His peace will come to you and that He will help you through each and every trial you may face in your life. May you have a long and happy life filled with many of God's rich blessings that He is so ready to bestow on you.

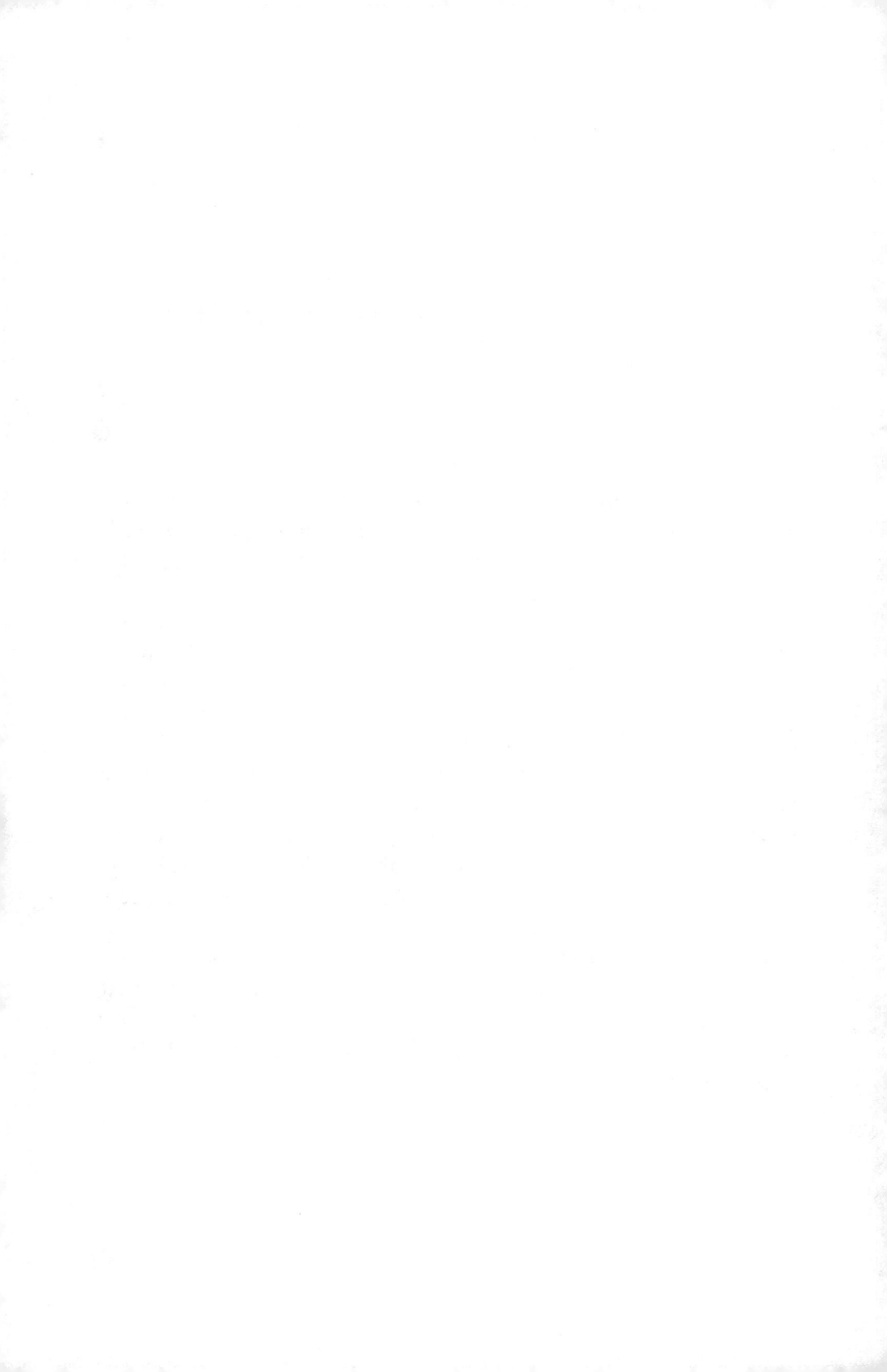

CHAPTER 1
A Seed Of Faith Was Planted

*"Train a child up in the way he should go, and when he
is old he will not depart from it".*

Proverbs 22:6

I was born in 1950 in Meridian, Mississippi to two wonderful people, Rev. Roy and Thelma Suitor. I was raised in Highland Methodist Church which was only about three blocks from our first home until I was around nine years old. We moved when I was in the third grade to the Northwest area of Meridian but we still attended Highland Methodist Church because it was still a short distance from our home. I was told just last week that my old "home" church, Highland Methodist is being sold now, which makes me have a sad feeling.

My parents had me baptized on Palm Sunday, which was the Sunday before Easter and I was just a few months old. I think just about every Palm Sunday since I was old enough to understand anything, my mother has told me about that baptism. She was so proud to have her daughter, the baby of the family, baptized on a special day like Palm Sunday.

My mom and dad took me to church every service, Sunday morning, Sunday night and Wednesday night. I was involved in the youth group MYF on Sunday evening before the church service at night. Some of my fondest memories now are of the friends I had at that church and the fun we had in Sunday School and MYF. I never realized that you could have so much fun and be learning about your Lord at the same time.

1

Children who are not taken to church miss out on so much. Rearing a child in church is one of the most important things you can do for them and I am so thankful to God that I had parents that realized that.

I am thankful also that they were parents that took me to church and didn't just drop me off there or send me with someone else. Them being there had a great influence on me and my life. They taught me that prayer was so important in life and then faith in God to answer those prayers was just as important. I remember praying when I was very small and believing in God to answer those prayers. My parents planted that seed within me to pray and believe and it has grown over the years tremendously.

My brother and his wife Peggy, were trying desperately to have a child when they first married. I was around fifteen years old at the time. I remember Peggy calling my mother and telling her that she wanted me to pray that she would be able to conceive a baby, they had been trying for so long with no luck. I began praying to God to bless Richard and Peggy with a child and the next thing we knew she had conceived her child that same month. That just reinsured me that there was indeed a God and He was waiting, listening and willing to answer my prayers whether small or large requests. It also made me feel good that Peggy had faith in my prayers. She knew that I had prayed all of my life and had so many prayers answered.

Do you know that God longs for us to talk to Him. He waits ever so patiently while we stay so busy in life that we do good to just say a nighttime prayer as we finish our day and turn in for the night. You know as I grew up and got oh, so busy, with whatever we get involved with, work, marriage, raising our family, I found myself praying less sometimes. I did good to say my bedtime prayers and so many times I would fall asleep while saying them. I would think a lot about how sad God must be that we get too busy to talk to Him. I think of all He has done for us and we can't or don't give Him anymore time than we do. But you know once a seed has been planted, such as the seed my parents planted in me, it grows and it stays with you. So, please teach your children to pray and believe and depend on God because it will carry them through every situation in their lives. "Train up the child in the way he should go and when he is old he will not depart from it".   (Proverbs 22:6)

I thank God for the seed planted in me and as you will see later in this book it has carried me through my breast cancer!

CHAPTER II
My Dad's Call To The Ministry

"Blessed is the man whom thou choosest, and causest to approach unto thee, that he may dwell in thy courts; we shall be satisfied with the goodness of thy house, even of thy holy temple."

Psalm 65:4

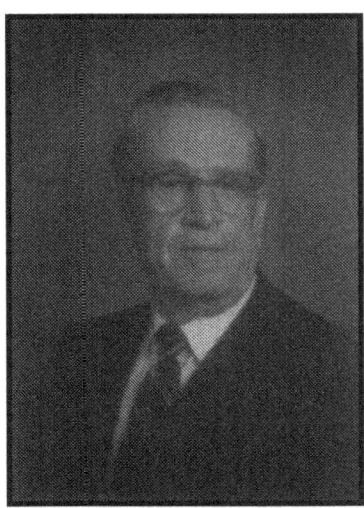

Cathy's dad-the late Rev. Roy Suitor

As a teenager I was still involved in Highland Methodist Church. Little did I know that God had called my daddy to preach many, many years earlier - before my birth even. My daddy, for different reasons, had not heeded the call. As the years had gone by dad felt sad and regretted not heeding the call from God to preach and he was getting up in years now and felt it was just too late to start preaching. Of course, the old devil was working on daddy and doing everything he could to convince him that it was indeed too late and that he had waited too long to become a preacher. Who in the world would want a sixty year old preacher just starting out in the ministry, inexperienced in the ministry at that. But God knows what He is doing. Remember?

5

Well one morning daddy woke up and the scripture Philippians 4:13 came to him which said "I can do all things through Christ which strengthens me". He jumped up and told my mother to get ready they were going to talk to the District Superintendent the Methodist Conference about daddy going into the ministry. They did meet with him that morning and the ball got rolling.

Daddy studied and completed whatever courses were required to become a preacher and passed with flying colors, which amazed him because he thought he was too old to go back to school. But God had a plan for Roy Suitor and He helped him all the way to complete what had to be done to accomplish God's plan.

Needless to say I was happy for daddy but sad that I would have to leave my church that I had attended all of my fifteen years of life. I had to leave not only Highland Methodist Church but also my friends there as we began daddy's ministry at Pleasant Grove Methodist Church in Kemper County. I made new friends however at that charge and soon became accustomed to being a "preacher's kid". I have always made a joke that they always say that preachers' kids are so bad but since my daddy didn't start preaching until I was fifteen years old I was only "half bad". (smile)

I had taken piano lessons for a few years and this came in handy when daddy needed someone to fill in for the regular piano player. In later years I became the full time pianist/organist at his last church. I was glad to play the piano and organ because I sure couldn't sing and would much rather play the piano than let anyone hear my voice singing. Daddy preached at Pleasant Grove Charge for two years and the people accepted him so well and were so happy to have him even if he was an elderly man. If you knew my daddy you know what a special person he was. He was a humble man and definitely lived what he preached. God does know who to call as his servants, and I believe God prepares them for service all along during their life. Mother told me that when my daddy was a child that he said he was so shy that if he was sitting in a room full of people that were at the house visiting, he would want to get up and go outside to play but was too shy to even get up and walk across the room in front of those visitors. Can you imagine someone like that ever standing in the pulpit and speaking in front of people.

Then in later years my daddy worked for Kraft Food Company as field manager which required him to speak in front of people which helped build the confidence he needed to fulfill God's plan for his later years. Daddy had also worked for Sears for twenty years and served as their Credit Manager which meant he had to deal with all types of people. Daddy always felt like the experience he had with Sears in dealing with people also better equipped him for future years when he would become a minister. My daddy had no idea that God was working all of this out in his life to prepare him for the ministry. You will see later in this book how God has done the same thing in my life and if you look back at your own life you can see how God has worked in your life to prepare you for certain situations. He is truly amazing. How can anyone deny the fact that there is a God?

After serving the Pleasant Grove Charge for two years daddy moved further to northern Kemper county to the Cleveland Charge. He was pastor for five churches within this charge. (Big Oak, Clarks Chapel, Shiloh, Mt. Pleasant, and Hopewell). Again we made many friends there and they too accepted daddy and our family so well. His age did not bother them at all. Daddy was not only a preacher but also a "pastor". He not only watched after his flock which was contained within five churches within that charge but he visited all the hospitals in Dekalb and Meridian, Miss. And visited people in the hospital that weren't even his members. He just wanted to let them know he cared and prayed with them. I must say that God blessed our family with so many wonderful people in the congregations at the churches he served.

Daddy was getting up in years now and felt that he needed to move back to the home place in Meridian to get my mother settled before he died. Sadly we left the Cleveland Charge. Many tears were shed that final day at that charge. I appreciate so much how well my daddy and our family were treated by all the churches he served but serving for thirteen and a half years in one church you really have a bond with the congregation.

Daddy was still able to preach and after he got settled back in Meridian in the home place he took an assignment to preach at

Cokers Chapel Methodist Church in Southeast Meridian. Again many wonderful people were there and we loved them too. Daddy was beginning to plan to retire since he was in his late seventies by now. But he was asked to take one more church. He agreed and began preaching at Hawkins Memorial Methodist Church.

Now at Hawkins Memorial Methodist Church I eventually became the full time pianist/organist due to the elderly organists death. I loved playing for them and they were always wonderful to me. This would be the last church for daddy to serve. He had planned to retire one day.

It wouldn't be but a couple of years before daddy's heart began to wear out. He had already had a pace maker inserted in his chest in order to survive. We eventually ended up in Jackson, Mississippi where tests were done that showed that daddy would probably not live over a year. I was devastated to say the least. To lose my daddy was an unbearable thought. I just didn't think I could go through giving my daddy up here on earth. But God will see you through anything if you will only depend on Him.

My daddy was a minister for twenty years before his death in 1986. So even though he didn't heed the call of God in his younger life, God never gave up on seeing his plan through. He knew Roy Suitor was the man for the job and He did not leave him alone until he took that call and then the Lord blessed not only my daddy with twenty years of life to win souls for Him, but he also blessed all of the people that daddy served all of those years.

Now, I have told you all of that to tell you this - - I wouldn't take anything in this world for being that "preachers' kid". He and my mother not only planted the seed but watered that seed with the wonderful life we had in the ministry.

CHAPTER III

My Mom's Trials Were Lessons For Me

"God is our refuge and strength, a very present help in trouble"

Psalms 46:1

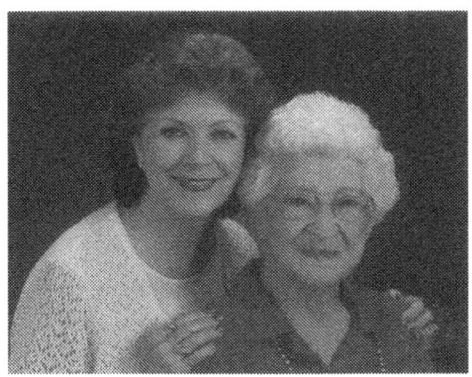

Cathy's 89 yr. old mom and Cathy during Cathy's journey with Breast cancer

I was taught all of my life that God never puts more on us than we can stand or that He is willing to carry us through. You can't help but question that sometimes and wonder how you would cope with trials when they come, and believe me, trials will come.

Trials surely come not only because we have the devil walking among us but also God allows trials to come to make us strong and to make us draw nearer to Him and to get us in a place He desires for us to be. I'll discuss exactly what I mean later in this book.

My mom has always been a strong woman in my eyes. She stood by my daddy in his ministry and even worked alongside him visiting the sick and shut-ins. Daddy always called her his "Associate Pastor" which I thought was so sweet.

One of the biggest trials I saw my mom go through was the sudden death of my brother, Richard, who died suddenly of a massive heart attack. Richard had not felt well for a while and was pale. He made an appointment with his doctor. On Saturday before his appointment on Tuesday he told his friends he felt like he was having a heart attack. He held his chest. They asked him if he wanted something to drink and he drank some ice water, which was probably the wrong thing to do because the cold drink probably made his arteries constrict. He got in a truck with his friend. The friend was driving, luckily. He said that Richard never spoke a word but fell over in his lap. He said that when he looked down into Richard's face he knew that he was gone. He drove straight to the hospital and Richard was pronounced dead on arrival. Richard was only 45 years old. So young....He was living in St. Petersburg, Florida at the time of his death.

I received the call from St. Petersburg, Florida from my nephew, Richard's son, that my brother was gone. I knew that I had to go to mother's and daddy's and break the horrible news to them that Richard was gone. How could I do this to them?

We had already been told that daddy was going to die within a year because of his failing heart. It was so hard telling them that Richard was gone. It was a beautiful sunny Saturday with a great breeze blowing. My daddy was having to wear nitroglycerin patches fo his heart/chest pains. When I arrived at the house mother and daddy were sitting in the back yard enjoying the beautiful day. I'll never forget that day as long as I live. When I told them daddy never moved but huge tears just rolled down his face.

Mother got up and began wandering aimlessly over the back yard in disbelief of what I had just told her. We all went inside the house and daddy went to his room and began changing his patches for his heart. Mother picked up a picture of Richard that was on her bedside table and began saying over and over, "Do you mean I will never see that pretty smile he had anymore?"

I thought sure that I was going to lose not only my brother that day but both of my parents too.

Somehow, and we all know how, my mother survived this terrible loss. She lost so much weight and cried many tears. How do you bury your child? But God took her hand and led her safely through this trial. I watched and learned a lot from my mother through this difficult trial. God did sustain her!

Then before she could recover from the loss of her son God called my daddy home to be with Him. My daddy's doctor called me one day at work and told me that he thought that I ought to know that after examining my daddy on his last checkup that he felt daddy didn't have much longer. I asked how long did he think? Dr. Carter said maybe three weeks.

It hurt to hear this news but I am so thankful that Dr. Carter took out time to call me and give me the "heads up" so that mother and I could prepare for the inevitable and tell daddy any and everything that we needed to tell him before he left this world.

I wrote daddy poems and I knew that he knew how much I loved him. I know my mother said her goodbyes to him in her own way too. Even though you think you are prepared, you never really are. One Saturday, sure enough about three weeks later, I drove toward mother and daddy's house. I was going up Highway 45 toward Meridian and passed a peach stand with two young boys working it. I thought "you know daddy loves peaches". I turned the car around and went back to that peach stand and bought daddy some peaches. I am so glad that I made that stop because when I arrived at my parents my mother met me in the hall and said that daddy wasn't doing well. I took his peaches to his room where he was lying on the bed. He was able to eat a few. The next day, Sunday, he got worse and I could see him rubbing his ankles together as he lay on the bed and I knew he was in a lot of pain. Daddy has never complained. When I went to him and asked if he was hurting bad he said "bad enough". I told him I wished he would let me call an ambulance so that he could go to the hospital so they could at least ease his pain. He finally agreed, though I know he would rather die in his own bed at home, but I just wanted some relief from pain for him.

I called the ambulance and told the dispatcher that my daddy was in congestive heart failure. I rode in the ambulance with daddy, which is right where he wanted me, and I sat in the emergency room with him with both of us knowing that his life here on earth was nearing an end.

After going to his room they did get daddy some relief and he could visit with us. He whistled for my daughter, Karen, who was nine years old at that time, which he always had done since she was big enough to walk.

He would whistle and point to his cheek and she would run over to him and kiss him on that cheek. So as always, this day was no different. She ran to the hospital bed and planted a big kiss on his right cheek. He smiled and his eyes sparkled. Oh how he loved my little girl and she loved him. I'm so thankful for my daddy and the wonderful grandfather he was to my daughter. She will never forget him and I am so glad she knew him. Soon we told daddy bye and I told him that I would take off from work the next day, Monday, and stay at the hospital with him.

I kissed him bye and left the hospital. About 10:30 P.M. that same night my mother called from the hospital and said that dad was worse. We went immediately to the hospital and found my mother outside of the hospital room in the hallway. A code 9 had been called and they were trying to resusitate my daddy. I stood outside the hospital room in the hallway and pleaded with God to please let my daddy come back long enough for me to tell him good bye. It seemed like an eternity but they finally rolled his bed, with him in it, out of the room and down the hall to the Cardiac Care Unit. His eyes were closed. I ran behind them all of the way to the CCU.

Shortly they came out and told us that we could go in and see daddy in CCU. I told mother to go first. She went in and talked with him. He had a tube in his mouth and was trying very hard to tell mother something. We have always wondered what he was trying to tell her. When mother came out of CCU I walked in to see daddy. Upon entering the room I could see that daddy was struggling to breathe. But when he saw me he layed back in the bed as if nothing was wrong. He did not want to upset me. He always thought of others and this time was no different. During the very last minutes of his life, the very end of his life, he was, as usual, thinking of others.

I hugged daddy and told him I loved him. He tried to tell me he loved me too but the tube in his mouth wouldn't let him speak.

Large tears rolled down his cheeks, not only because he knew he was leaving, but also because he was unable to say anything to me. I began to cry and daddy's eyes shifted to look at the nurse. He knew that she would make me leave the room if she thought my crying would upset him. I patted him on the chest and told him I would "see him later" and I believe that he knew as well as I did that I meant I would see him later in Heaven. He and I both knew it was his time to go to be with the Lord. I left that room knowing that once again God had answered my prayer by allowing daddy to return from the brink of death long enough to let me say my last farewell and now my second prayer would be outside the CCU and it would be this - "God if my daddy can't breathe and he is suffering, please do no let him linger and suffer - take him home to be with you now". And God immediately answered my prayer and took my daddy to his heavenly home where he finally sat at Jesus' feet and experienced true peace and was warmed by the love of God. My second prayer that night anwered by a true and faithful God. My God, My Friend.

This was a trial for my mother, my daughter and I but again God carried us through. My mother was so lost at the house without my daddy. God gave her the strength day by day and she became even stronger in the Lord. I continued to watch and learn from my sweet mother and her trials.

There were two more deaths to come soon. One was my sister, Peggy, who died from cancer and then second brother, Paul (we called him Buddy), who died on the operating table while having heart surgery. Two more children for my mother to bury. That would be a total of three children and a husband that my mother buried within two years. How do you go through losing a child, much less three children in two years and a mate? Only God could see you through that. He IS where our strength comes from. I continued to watch and learn.

Mother continued to age. She was very active and smiled and continued to witness to others just by how she handled all of her trials. People were absolutely amazed at her strength. She has always given God all of the credit for seeing her through everything.

Then in 1999 I got the call that my last sibling, a brother, Jimmy, had died exactly like my first brother Richard. Jimmy was having chest pains and sweating profusely. He lived in Jackson, Mississippi at this time. He stopped at a friends house and when he arrived at their door they asked him if he was alright. He was so pale and sweating. He told them he didn't feel well and they brought him in and had him sit on the couch. They offered him something to drink. He took some orange juice and they said that he took one sip and fell over on the couch. He was dead from a massive heart attack just like Richard died from in 1985. After receiving the call from Jimmy's wife that he was gone I immediately thought of his daughter Lori and his son, Johnny and my mother. I was going to have to let all of them know this horrible news. I called Betty, who is Lori and Johnny's mother. Johnny was living out of town at the time. Lori worked at Medical Towers in Meridian. Betty called Lori's husband, Charles and together they went to Lori's work and called her to come downstairs. When she saw her mother and husband together and looked at their face she said that she just knew something had happened to her daddy. She was devastated, as was her brother, Johnny.

Then I had to once again go to my mother's house and tell her that another one of her children had died. She said then that she hoped that she would never have to bury me, her daughter and the baby of the family and the only child she had left. She said she just didn't think that she could go through that. Now if I ever had a doubt that God would not put more on you than you could stand all doubt was erased. Because I learned a great lesson through my mother's trials and that was that whatever trials God allows to happen in our lives He is more than willing to carry us through victoriously to the other side of that trial.

As the famous poem states, God told us that when we saw only one set of footprints "it is then that I carried you". That is so true when you look back at your life. Look back at yours and see how he carried you through when you couldn't carry yourself.

CHAPTER IV
Where Does The Time Go?

"But this I say, brethren, the time is short"

I Corinthians:7:29

You know when you look back on your life you wonder where the time went? The childhood years, teens, young adult hood and before you know it you are in your forty's.

I had my daughter, Karen, eight years after getting married. At first I wanted to wait a while and enjoy being married first and have children later. Then as the years went by I realized I was in my late twenties and I needed to begin a family. We tried to conceive for a long while, but to no avail. Finally God answered our prayers and I conceived a little baby.

The entire time I carried my child I prayed to God, in detail, about just how I wanted her to look. Features that I didn't like about myself I prayed she would not have and features I liked about her daddy I prayed she would have. I prayed that she would have her daddy's eyes, nose and complexion especially - and yes, God answered those prayers to a tee.

I thought I wanted a little boy the whole time I was pregnant. I guess I thought most men want a son to carry on their name. I picked out a boys name but would not pick out a girls name because "I wasn't having a girl". I was going to name my boy "Eric Randall". About two weeks before the birth of my child my husband said I should pick out a girls name just in case it was a girl. So, I decided to name a girl (just in case it was a girl) "Karen Lowetta". My middle name was Lowetta. This name had been used all through the family.

My mother had the name Lowetta, my cousin did and one of my twin nieces did.

Well, the day came that my child was born and yes, it was a girl. When they brought her to the head of the bed for me to see her I couldn't have been happier that she was in fact a girl.. How could I have ever wanted a little boy? She was beautiful and had an olive complexion and dark hair all over her little head.

I enjoyed so much having a little girl. All the fun things we did and the stuffed animals that I bought for her, but a lot of times I bought them because deep down I was still a little girl and loved stuffed animals. My daughter also had a little tom boy in her and I'm glad of that too. She liked to fish, ride four wheelers, and could hold her own with the boys if they picked on her.

There are so many memories of her childhood but one of the cutest things she said once was when she was about three years old she was standing barefoot on the couch looking over the bar at me while I was cooking supper. All of a sudden she said "there is a mouse". We were in our new house and

I had never seen a mouse in there before. I quickly looked at her and asked, "Karen, are you telling a story?" Without missing a beat she said, "once upon a time there was a mouse". Her interpretation of "story" was not that she was telling a fib but that she was telling a little storybook story. You are probably like me, you could never name all the memories you have of your children. One more I have is when Karen was about two years old and I dressed her up in a beautiful pink Easter dress and frilly bonnet. Remember now that she has a little tom boy in her. We headed to church and before we got to the church she had pulled that bonnet off of her head. I put it back on her head and by the time we walked up to the front porch of the church I looked down at her and she had that bonnet off again. I once again put the bonnet back on her head and we walked down the aisle of the church. By the time we got seated in the pew I looked at her and she had taken that bonnet off of her head again. Needless to say I gave up on her wearing the bonnet...

Before you know it Karen is grown up and dating and getting married. She looked absolutely beautiful in her wedding dress with the heart cut out in the back of the dress.

I have watched that video and looked at the wedding pictures a million times, at least. Where does the time go?

The next thing you know my baby is going to have a baby of her own? I am going to be a grandmother? Are you kidding? I'm too young for that…Well, not really, I was about 45 years old. Older than I think.

Karen and I figured she was having a little girl that whole time she was pregnant. My mother, Karen's Big Mom, said all along that it would be a boy. Never underestimate the "Vibes" of a great-grandmother. Because sure enough Karen had a little boy. I couldn't have been happier and Karen and her husband couldn't have been happier to have a boy.

They made it a joint effort to name him. One picked out the name, "Cody" and the other picked out the name "Lane" so they had a Cody Lane. I have always been told that there is nothing like grandchildren, and that is so true. It is wonderful to have a grandchild because your child is in that child also.

And as I keep saying, God knows just what He is doing. I had only one child, a daughter and she had a son; so I tell her that she was my girl and she had me a little boy to enjoy. Now I got to experience taking care of a little girl and a little boy. I thank God for that too.

I have been blessed so much by my God in my lifetime and if we all take time to look back at our life we can see the miracles God has worked in our lives as well as the road map that He went by to guide and direct us in the paths He wanted us to take. Yes, sometimes we waiver and we get off of the path. I went astray many times, and just because my daddy was a preacher doesn't mean I am without sin, or perfect. No one is perfect. I believe that the more we try to live and work for God the harder the devil works to draw us away from God. That has been true in my life.

The most wonderful thing about God is that He is a forgiving God. All we have to do is ask for forgiveness for our sins and He forgives gladly. Once forgiven we strive even harder to do better and steer away from sin. He is a loving and forgiving God.

About nine months after Cody was born my husband and I decided we would retire from our job at East Miss. State Hospital.

We had enough time to retire. I was given a wonderful retirement party at the hospital and I have wonderful memories of that day also. I was allowed to make a talk and my former boss, Vince, made a speech that brought tears to everyone's eyes, including mine. He has a real talent for speaking and also being humorous. As a matter of fact he was always downright hilarious.

We enjoyed retirement so much. You don't have to worry about setting an alarm clock and getting up day after day to go to work. I got to enjoy being with my little peek-a-pooh dog who had spent so much time at home alone while we worked. He was like another child. His name was Truman and he was definitely one of the family. We bought us a camper and began camping some and that was fun for us also. Although, I told my husband that really campers are for people that live in town or a heavily populated place that need to get away from it all. Our house was down in the woods in the country and we were already away from it all; but we did enjoy the experience of camping for a while.

The next thing you know Karen has decided to go back to work because Cody is fourteen months old now. My husband said that since we were retired there was no reason Cody should have to go to day care, we could baby-sit him. I really appreciated him for that. It not only allowed us to be with Cody a lot but it kept his parents from having to pay for expensive child care. We couldn't have been happier keeping that precious little boy.

We felt like Cody was the little boy we didn't have. We would take him swimming in the pool, fishing, riding the four wheeler, playing ball, you name it we did it. We watched that little boy grow up and start to school. We babysat him after school too and he spent the night with us a lot. I only regret that I didn't get to spend as much time with my own daughter when she was a child but these days it takes both parents working to make a living so I worked all of her childhood just like she is having to do with Cody.

Well, the next thing I know my daughter has decided to take a new job and move to Florida. By now Cody is seven years old. You can imagine how attached we are to Cody and how accustomed we are to having him around. Needless to say we were devastated to hear she and Cody were moving away. My immediate thought was how far away is that and how fast can I get there if I need to get there? I got out a map and that didn't mean a lot to me. I got Cody in the car the next weekend and drove to see how long it would take to get to their new location. It took me three hours. "Well, that's not as bad as I thought it would be", I thought. I started praying a lot for God to please help me with this adjustment in my life and to please bless my precious angels, Karen and Cody. I thought my world was coming apart at the seams. I realize people have their children and grandchildren living in far off places and it doesn't seem like a big deal but to me at this particular time it was. I had wrapped myself all up into Cody. He was the very center of my life. Looking back I realize that maybe I was too wrapped up in him. But I am still thankful to God for all of those years that I did get to spend so much time with Cody and share good times with him. I believe he will always cherish the memories of being at "memaws and papas"......

As it turned out Karen had to work a lot at night when she first moved to Florida and day cares close at 6PM. Being retired I was able to go with her to Florida and keep Cody after school each day since she didn't get home till late at night.

I would stay every week and Cody and I would come to Mississippi on the weekends so I could see my husband, then we would head back on Sunday night. I did this for about four months until we finally found a lady in town that we could hire to keep Cody after school and until Karen got off work at night.

I have always made a joke and told people that I was so upset that Karen and Cody were moving that I just moved with them....It all worked out fine though and I finally adjusted to being away from Cody some. However, I did travel every other weekend and bring him to visit Mississippi. Cody is almost ten years old now and they have been in Florida for three years and God has blessed me through the adjustment and all of the traveling.

But, as I said before - - - Where does the time go? What do we do with our time? I was always told that the older you get the faster the time goes and I have found that to be true.

Now it was the year 2005 and I had been traveling, as usual, every other weekend to pick Cody up and bring him to Mississippi. Time was really going by fast now. It seemed like Cody had grown up so fast. When he stood next to me his head reached my chin. I would soon be looking up at him.

My mother's little peek-a-pooh, named Baby-Doll, looked so much like my little peek-a-pooh, Truman. We always said that if they hadn't had surgery we would have loved to have seen them have puppies. They would have been so cute. Mother's little baby-doll was old, just like Truman now. We found a knot on baby-doll's breast area. It was growing. I took her to the Vet, Dr. Donaldson, and she said that mother's little pet had a tumor. She steadily got worse. Dr. Donaldson said that as long as we could keep baby-doll comfortable and she would eat, we could put off having her put to sleep. I wanted to put it off as long as possible because baby-doll was so much company for my mother since she lived alone. Mother took good care of baby-doll and her little pet seemed to be comfortable and was eating well. So we waited....

Then during the summer, June, 2005, Truman, my little peek-a-pooh, began running into the furniture. He would get up into a corner and couldn't figure out how to back out. I didn't know what in the world was wrong with him.

We had bought Truman when he was a puppy and he was now 13 years old. (A little old man) He was a lap dog for sure. He never weighed over 10 pounds. If I was sitting in my chair, he was in my lap. He slept in our bed with us at night. He was just one more member of our family, just like another child. I was way too attached to him. What in the world was wrong with my little dog?

He was pitiful. He acted like he had gone blind. I would hold him and he would stretch his legs out and hollar. The veterinarian was closed so I toughed it out all night with him. I noticed that he would walk along and just fall over. When he would hollar I thought something was hurting or he was being eaten up on the inside. I thought of everything....

Morning couldn't come soon enough. My husband and I got dressed and carried Truman to the Vet. I was so emotional I couldn't even talk to the receptionist. I just held him in my arms, wrapped in a blanket; then she came and got me and guided me back to the doctors. Dr. Daniel Newell looked at him and immediately told me that it looked as if Truman had a stroke. I hadn't even thought about "stroke", even though I do know that it can cause blindness and paralyses, and neurological problems. Now I understood why he couldn't see, would fall over and couldn't figure out how to back out of a corner....The doctor went on to say, "you know what we need to do?" I said, "yes, I would have done it last night if I could have, just to get him out of his misery." I chose to stay in the room while they gave Truman the shot that put him to sleep. I told Truman bye and kept my hand on him so that he would know that I was with him until the end. He was faithful to me all of his little life and I was determined to be there for him. That was a very hard day for me. Another trial. Bob and I brought him home and we buried him up on the hill by our house.

My daughter, Karen, bought a beautiful tomb stone with a beautiful poem engraved on it. Truman was bought for Karen when she was a teenager but she allowed me to keep him when she married. Thank God, because Truman helped with my "empty nest syndrome" after Karen moved away. Now, our Truman was gone to the other side. Bye my faithful friend, I love you......

Well, it wasn't a month later that my mother's dog began getting worse. She now had many knots all over her abdomen. It was hard for us to touch her without it hurting her. Mother and I knew it was time to take her to the vet and get her out of her misery. It broke my mothers heart that day when I came to pick baby-doll up. It broke mine too. I loved that little dog and she always clung to me when I came for a visit to mothers. I would miss her too. I could not believe that I was going to have to go through this again when I hadn't even had time to get over Truman yet. But I sure didn't want my mother to have to do it.

I took baby-doll, wrapped up in her little blanket, and headed out to the veterinarians. I took her in and Dr. Donaldson looked at her and agreed that it was time. I again, decided to stay in the room so that baby-doll would know I was there for her. Dr. Donaldson gave her the shot and baby-doll went easy just like Truman had. I also made sure that I told her good-bye and that I loved her before she left this world. I kept my hand on her until she was gone. Now we brought another little pet home to be buried on the hill.

There had been several bad things happen during this year "2005" and this was just two more. We are at the latter part of the summer now and I am saying, "This has been a terrible year, this year "2005", I wonder what else could happen?" Don't ever ask that question - because as you will see in the next chapter, it can get worse......

CHAPTER V
"It Couldn't Happen To Me:" Ignoring the Signs of Cancer"

"If thou faint in the day of adversity, thy strength is small"

Proverbs 24:10

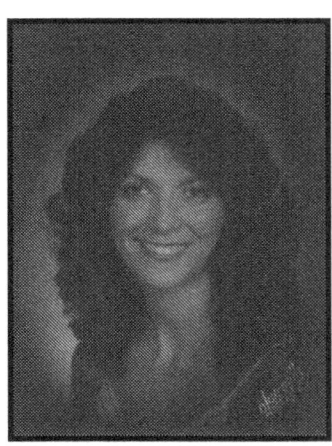

Cathy before breast cancer.

I believe we all feel that cancer is something that happens to everyone else. Even though my sister and my aunt had died from cancer I still did not ever think that I would have cancer. I took vitamins regularly and I didn't smoke, drink or do drugs. The only drug problem I had ever had is that my parents drug me to church every time the church doors were open. I never knew I could be so proud of any one fact than I am of that. I am so thankful they did drag me to church and teach me about God, prayer and faith because those teachings have seen me through some difficult times in my life. What do people do without God in their life? It would be impossible to make it on your own - you can't......

For a while I had been noticing a knot in my left breast. I was still running all the time and too busy to really think about it much. Anyway, the knot was in exactly the same spot where a knot had been removed about eleven years earlier that proved to be benign. I was very worried when that first knot was removed and I prayed so hard about it and was so thankful when the tests proved it to be benign. I thanked God over and over.

There couldn't be anything wrong.

My Fear That Something Was Wrong:

Well, I continued to run back and forth to Florida. I noticed that I was more tired than usual and irritable too. I just contributed all of that to all of my traveling.

Now it was October, 2005. Again as I lay down one night to go to sleep I felt that ominous knot in my left breast. I wondered? Could there be something wrong? Some people say if it hurts it is not cancer and some say if it doesn't hurt it isn't cancer. Which is it? All kinds of questions were sweeping through my mind. I felt so scared and so uncertain, yet I still had a peace that I could not have cancer. Not me.

The next morning I got out of bed and when I was in the bathroom getting ready I noticed "dimpling" in my left nipple. I thought, "Oh, No". I could also feel what felt like a knot in the lower part of the nipple. I immediately went to the den and showed my husband. He looked at me and said there is a knot there. I said, "I know, I think I need to call and get my mammogram appointment soon."

I got to thinking that maybe something was wrong. You know children are very perceptive and it hadn't been but a few weeks since my grandson, Cody was spending the night with me and we went to bed one night and he put his little arms around my neck and pulled me up really close to him and said, "Memaw, I don't know what I would do if anything ever happened to you." Was this a premonition?

Also, Cody sat down in the recliner with me one night after I found the knot in my breast. He accidentally bumped my left side and I told him, "be careful baby, Memaw has a knot in her breast. That precious little boy turned and looked me straight in the eyes and said, "you probably have breast cancer". Could I? Where had he heard that? Then I remembered it was October and it was "Breast Cancer Awareness Month" and there had been a lot on television about that. Maybe that was just a coincidence that he knew about something like that....

I called my family physician and asked if I could get a mammogram appointment made and also an appointment to see her. The earliest mammogram appointment they could get me would be December. They said I could come in for my annual exam with the doctor the latter part of the next week. I now had two appointments. One with my doctor for the next week and one for a mammogram for December. This was on Friday when I called.

By the following Monday I noticed a knot had developed under my left arm. I knew that this was not a good thing. I immediately remembered that your lymph nodes are in different areas of your body and one place is under your arms.

My sister had cancer in 1986 and was told it had spread to her lymph nodes and she had six months to live. She survived a little longer - one year....

Needless to say, I thought about Peggy when I had the swollen lymph node under my arm. My fear was real, "What if I have Cancer?" I couldn't get past that thought, I couldn't even think about anything else, such as my family. The same thought just kept ringing over and over in my head, "what if I have cancer?"

I ran to the phone and called my family physician's office again and told them that I had found an additional knot and it was under my left arm and "I needed to come in to see the dr. today". They were very nice and told me to come on in that afternoon.

Before going to the doctor I had called my friend, Diane, who had been diagnosed with breast cancer three years earlier. I'll never forget the day that I heard she had breast cancer. Diane and I were friends from birth and had lived in the same neighborhood, by Highland Park, until I was in the third grade and we moved to Northwest Meridian. I didn't get to see her as much after moving away because we were at different schools. As the years went by though we found each other again. Diane's mother was diagnosed with breast cancer and the doctor gave her absolutely no hope of living because he saw a "dimple" in her breast. She however did have the mastectomy and chemo and the whole nine yards and she lived eleven more years. The cancer eventually returned and spread to her bones then her brain. It breaks your heart to listen to Diane describe the latter part of her mothers illness and eventual death. Sometimes death can be a relief and I believe it was in her moms case, bless her heart.

Now it was 2003 and I was at my mother's house getting ready to go to church with her for Easter Sunday. I was in the kitchen and my mother had just gotten the Sunday newspaper. She called me to come there and told me that it was on the front page - an article telling that my friend, Diane, had been diagnosed with breast cancer.

It told about her surgery and what she had gone through. All I could do was cry. It hadn't been that long since I had been over at Diane's house. It had all happened so fast. She was only a couple of months overdue for her mammogram when her daughter prompted her to get an appointment to check her breasts. Diane did go and the next thing she knew she was told she had breast cancer. They did a radical mastectomy and reconstruction of her breasts at the same time. They had found it early enough so that they did not feel it necessary for her to have chemotherapy nor radiation. I was thankful for that, but I still could not help but cry because I thought I was going to lose my friend and that she was going to die. Even early stage cancer can return and get you..... I will never forget the sadness I felt that day and how helpless I felt to help Diane. I did do a lot of praying, however, because I do believe in prayer.

But now back to the day I found the knot under my arm and I called Diane. I called to ask her what she thought about my symptoms. You know you reach out for any and everybody you can to advise you or give you some hope. Diane said that she knew of cases sometimes when lymph nodes would swell like that due to a "cat scratch". Boy was I relieved because my grandson's cat had "scratched off" on my leg a couple of weeks before this time and I had some deep bloody scratches on

my legs. This was welcome news to my ears and I decided that I didn't have cancer I just had a reaction to that "cat scratch"...I know that Diane was hoping beyond hope that I didn't have cancer but I found out later from her that when I had told her about the dimpling in my nipple she was so afraid it was cancer. Of course she didn't say anything about it that day but I know that she did some hard praying for me then. She is a good, Christian friend.

I went on to the doctor that afternoon. I immediately mentioned the "cat scratch" possibility. Sure enough there had been a few of those cases recently, but my doctor informed me that this was not one of those cases. She checked my breasts and under my arm. She said she felt there was definitely "something going on in there".

She made an appointment for me with Dr. Sandra Pupa, a Radiologist, so that I could have a mammogram and go from there. Still I wondered, "Could I have Cancer?"

This is Monday and my appointment with Dr. Pupa would not take place until Thursday. It would make for a long two or three more days…

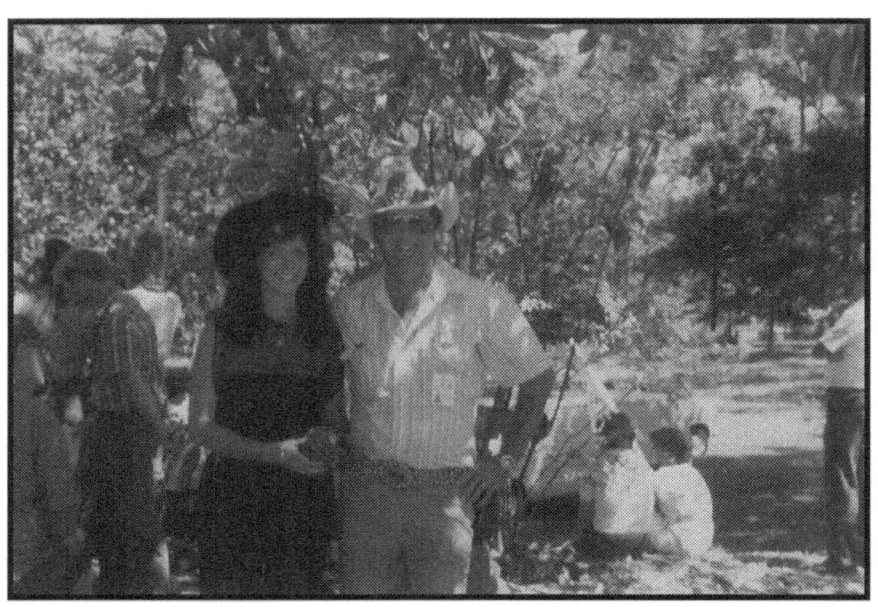

Cathy with husband, Bob, when first married, 1986.

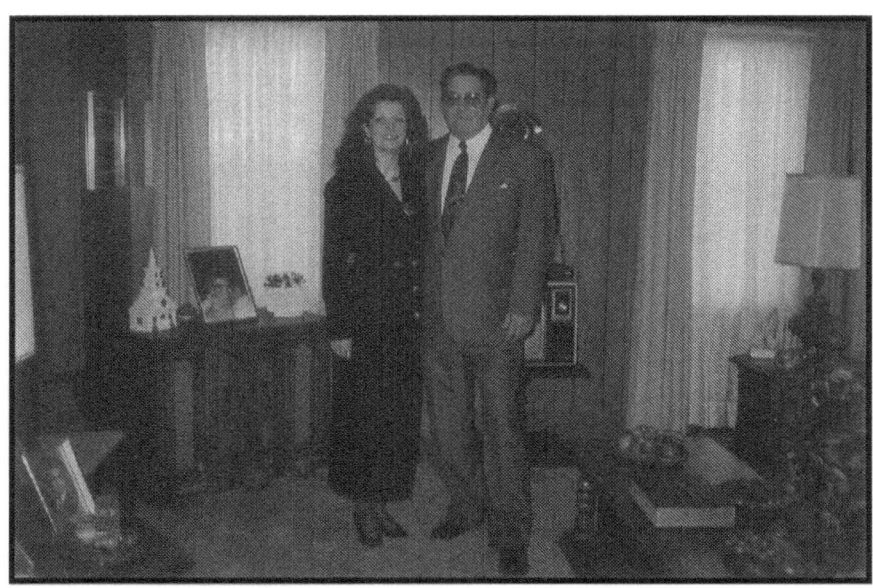

Cathy with husband, Bob, just before their retirement.

CHAPTER VI
Being Diagnosed with Breast Cancer

"I waited patiently for the Lord; and He inclined unto me, and heard my cry"

Psalms 40:1

The following Wednesday night I spoke with friends and family about what was going on with me and that I wanted them to all pray that my visit to the radiologist would prove that I did not have cancer. They were all reassuring and I knew that they were going to pray for my well being. That was a great sense of relief also and it got me through that night somehow.

The following day, Thursday, my husband and I drove to Dr. Sandra Pupa's office. She was a radiologist that I had never met. We sat in the waiting room and we both thumbed through magazines. I was barely able to concentrate on the magazine and couldn't help wondering if my husband was just going through the motions of thumbing through books also. I thought that like me, he probably had his mind on the "what ifs' of my situation.

Bob is nineteen years older than me. I couldn't help but think that I had always planned to be here to take care of him in his golden years. I surely didn't want or expect him to have to take care of me. "Oh, please dear Lord, don't let me have cancer and be a burden to everyone", I prayed silently.

In just a short time the receptionist called me to go in for the mammogram. It was pretty routine. They showed me to a small dressing area where I removed my top and bra and put on the little blue gown. Then I was led into the room with the big machine used for the mammogram.

The technician made all of the views of both of my breasts that she felt necessary. Still this was what I was use to experiencing annually. When she completed the pictures she took me to another room to await Dr. Pupa. As I looked around the room I saw information about mammograms, and other medical information, but what really caught my eye were the pictures, plaques and unique little things that were in that room that related to God and healing. That is a comforting feeling to know that these medical people know where their help comes from, as do I.

Before too long the door opened and an attractive, slim lady appeared and took my hand. She said, Cathy, my name is Sandi Pupa. I am going to let you go back over to the other room and let my technician make some more views of your breasts. She was so pleasant and friendly but I felt a little uneasiness inside me because why do they need more views? Did they see something bad? Do I have cancer? It is amazing how many thoughts can run through your mind in just a matter of seconds.

I tried to keep my composure and act like I wasn't worried. I'm sure Dr. Pupa has been around long enough to know that I was probably freaking out inside even if I didn't show it.

I went to the other room and the technician began taking more views. I did notice that she was a little shook up herself. She apologized for having to do more views because she couldn't remember which were which. I knew something must be wrong by her being so shook up. I really felt bad for her. She was such a sweet girl. Once she did complete that round of pictures she led me back to the examining room to wait again for Dr. Pupa.

Shortly Dr. Pupa came into the room. Again she took my hand, ever so sweetly, and looked me right in the eyes. She was pleasant, but concerned. She told me, and I'll never forget those words: "Cathy, there have been a lot of changes in both of your breasts since your last mammogram ten months ago".

I immediately blurted out, "both of my breasts?" She said, "yes". "How could it be in both my breasts?", I thought.

Dr. Pupa then explained that she was going to do a sonogram on both of my breasts. I was still in a daze. I laid down on the examining table and she put the cold gel on my breasts and began the sonogram. She showed me that I could watch on the little screen beside the bed. Once she had completed this sonogram she put the pictures up on the lighted board. She began pointing out tumor after tumor in both breasts. Now I was really scared. I knew that even if a woman had only one little bitty tumor in only one breast even, she could be in a real tough situation, a life threatening situation. Now I'm sitting here with several tumors in both breasts. My final day on this earth must be coming soon is all I could think.

In talking I mentioned my husband and she asked if he was with me. I told her he was in the waiting room. She said she would go get him. In a few minutes she returned with Bob following her. She said she didn't have any trouble finding him because he was the only man in the waiting room. I am so thankful he chose to go with me that day and I wasn't alone.

Dr. Pupa began showing him the pictures from the sonogram and explained to him that each of those black places were tumors. She told him that I had breast cancer and it was in both breasts. Bob looked as if he would burst into tears any moment, but managed somehow to hold it together. Dr. Pupa finally turned her back to me and looked Bob straight in the face and her words were, "it's bad news, but it could be worse". She told Bob to give me a hug. He leaned over and gave me a little hug and I apologized for having cancer. Dr. Pupa told him to give me a BIG hug, that women need those big hugs. So he did give me a big hug and told me we would be alright. He kept telling Dr. Pupa we would be alright, we would make it, but I wasn't too sure about that.

Dr. Pupa then told my husband he could wait in the waiting room while she did biopsies on both of my breasts to determine what type of cancer I had. She said that it would take longer just to prepare for the biopsies than to actually do them. She was right. She and her nurses draped me and prepared me. She explained exactly what it would sound like when she gathered the biopsy. Kind of like a staple gun going off. She told me I could watch the screen again while she did the biopsies. It is amazing what they can do medically these days. I was trying so hard to be brave and hold up. All I could think of is "I have cancer. I am going to die and leave my family behind. What will my nine year old grandson, Cody, do without his memaw? What will my eighty-eight year old mother do without me, her only child that is left on this earth? And, I thought I was going to live to be old and take care of Bob as he is getting older.....

As she began the biopsies my arms, hands and whole body began shaking uncontrollably. She thought I was cold but I told her no, I just can't quit shaking. Dr. Pupa then explained that when we are afraid and we can't run away that is how our body reacts. It was difficult for her to do the biopsy, I'm sure with me shaking so bad. Then as we all talked, trying to pretend everything was normal, I happened to see a picture on the wall of a small boy, and yes, I thought of my Cody. I began crying and the nurse brought me Kleenex. I wanted to be strong but I was so emotional. I hated it. I hate being out of control like that.

Once the biopsies were completed and labeled Dr. Pupa told me that I would need to return to her office the next day to find out what type of cancer I had. She had already told me that she felt that it was invasive and non-invasive ductal carcinoma. The word invasive, I knew was not good. I did not know a lot about cancer but I knew what invasive meant...

Dr. Pupa asked me what surgeon I would like to use because I would have to have a mastectomy. I had to try to find out what surgeon I would want to do that terrible surgery. (I couldn't even bare to think about that surgery yet) I was scheduled to return to her office the next day.

CHAPTER VII

*Breaking The News To My Family
And Friends*

*"Notwithstanding ye have well done, that ye did help
with my affliction"*

Philippians: 4:14

Bob and I somehow managed to walk to the car after this terrible ordeal. I told him I thought we should go straight to my mother's and tell her. She and my daughter had reassured me the night before that they were sure that everything was alright and that when I went to the doctor I would find out that nothing was wrong.

All of the way to mothers all I could think about was that she had buried her husband and four children and I was the baby of the family and the only child she had left. I could hear her voice over and over (after my last brother had died) saying, "Cathy, I hope I never have to bury you, I don't think I could bear that!" Now, how could I go and tell her that not only did I have breast cancer but I had breast cancer in both breasts. Dr. Pupa had told me that this is very rare for it to be in both breasts. I thought it must surely be spread all over my body if it is in both breasts already....My poor mom. What will she do. One thing I knew for sure was that she would not let me see her cry. She would stand strong and try to act like she was okay.

Well, we arrived at her house. My husband and I sat down with her in her den. I told her that I had just come from the

Radiologist's office and that I had breast cancer and it was in both breasts. No, she didn't cry. She stood strong just like I knew she would; but I will never, ever forget the look on her face that day. She looked just like someone had hit her square in the face with a board. She looked pale and it looked really as if her nose flattened for a moment just like a board had slammed her in the face. She did say she just couldn't believe it. When my husband and I drove off I told him that mom would go back in the house now and cry. I found out later she did. I asked her to call the church prayer list and get it started, because I knew I needed all the prayers I could get.

We got in the truck and decided we would go and get something to eat. On the way I called Florida to break the news to my precious daughter, Karen. She was scheduled to work late that day so she wouldn't be going to work until noon. I called her cell phone. When she answered I reminded her that I had been to the Radiologist. I told her that I had breast cancer. You could hear the shock in her voice. I went on to tell her that it was in both breasts and she began to cry. She had dated a boy when she was about sixteen and his mother had battled breast cancer for several years and ended up losing the battle. I was sure that she was thinking about that sad time and that she was scared that she, too, would lose her mother to this "mean" disease. A mother never wants her child to be sad or cry and the only thing I could think to say to her was "don't cry". What did I expect? I know I would cry if my mother told me that type of news. She told me later that she cried and cried and all she could think about was the fact that I was going to lose my hair and both of my breasts. She said she knew she wouldn't be able to cope with that if it were her that had the breast cancer.

I then decided that I should call my niece, Lori, because she goes to my mothers church and mother was going to have the prayer chain started for me and I didn't want Lori to hear about my cancer from anyone other than me. She is like another daughter to me. I made a call to her at work. She happens to work at the Anderson Cancer Center where they give chemotherapy and radiation. Just a few weeks before my diagnosis I had passed the Cancer Center and thought to myself, "I hope I never have to go to that place". Little did I know I would be going that soon....Lori was very emotional when I broke the news to her. She loves me and I love her. She would have to break the news to her family and her brother, Johnny, who is my nephew…(He was living out of town).

I then called my close friend, Jackie, that I had worked with at East Miss. State Hospital. She was so shocked. Even though I had asked her to pray the day before I went for testing, I believe she was like everyone else, she just thought it was going to be nothing.

We just talked a short time and later Jackie told me that she just didn't know what to say. I'm sure I would have been the same way if she had told me that kind of news about her…What do you say? What can you say? It is all so uncertain and so scary for everyone. I believe that Jackie has called me almost every day since I told her about my cancer. She has been so faithful to me. She put together a basket at East Miss. State Hospital and let friends donate gifts and cards to me. I received a lot of goodies in that basket. The body lotions, books, candles, candy, everything meant so much to me. God really blessed us when He gave us friends..

Bob and I got home and the next call I received was from my cousin, Lillian, who is like a sister to me. She and her husband, Bill have always been like an older brother and sister to me. She told me she was so sorry that I had received this bad news. They are very Christian people and I knew that they would be prayer warriors for me and that they would have their church and friends praying. She broke the news to my other family in her town. I have an Aunt Lillian there and a cousin Mike and his wife, Tereatha. They, too, all began praying for me and putting me on prayer lists. I called my cousin, Ann, in Jackson and she put me on the prayer list on the Internet and at churches. All these praying people give you some reassurance and hope…

My daughter called and said that she and Cody's daddy had discussed whether or not to tell Cody about my cancer yet. They decided that he would be asking questions when I started losing my hair and I would be losing my hair quickly if I had to have chemotherapy. She told Cody that night. He listened to her explain that I had breast cancer and then he told her, "I need to be alone for a few minutes" and he went to his bedroom and closed the door. I figure he may have cried and he probably prayed. We have taught him to pray about everything. I was worried about the toll this cancer would take on my whole family and especially a little nine year old boy. God Bless Him.

I began calling the different churches I had been attending so that everyone I knew could be praying for my healing. My pastor, Rev. Pam Randall, at Wesley Chapel Methodist Church, was so sad to hear my news. She wanted to come to me and hold me immediately, but she had no idea where my house was. She wanted directions to my house but I told her it was hard to find and we just planned to meet at the church one night. She sat with me while I talked about this terrible diagnosis, my fears, my family, and my hope in God. She cried with me, held my hand and read scriptures to me. I will never forget what a help she was to me and how she reached out to me. She is one of my encouragers and has been there for me the whole journey…She was my friend even before the diagnosis but we are even closer now I think. She is not only a wonderful preacher but a wonderful "pastor" and friend to her congregation.

Now you can probably guess that there was no sleep in the Riley household that night. I tried so hard to sleep but my mind wouldn't stop working and dwelling on the fact that now I know that "I DO HAVE CANCER". What now? I felt like I was caught in some kind of trap and had no way out. I was.

All I could think about was that I was to return to Dr. Pupa the next day to see "what kind of cancer" I had. That is what I thought Dr. Pupa had told me. Really it was an appointment to confirm the type of cancer she had already told me that I had, but I was so out of it I thought she was waiting to see what type I had.

Then Friday morning arrives and I feel terrible. I have had no sleep. I have cried and worried and prayed. Worried and prayed should not be in the same sentence because we are not suppose to worry. We are to pray and leave it in God's hands. That wasn't easy for me to do right now. I was feeling so desperate and alone. Yes, my husband was with me, but I still felt so alone and scared. There really was nothing he could do to help me.

I felt like I just wanted to go back in time and do something different; something that could change what was happening to me now. What if I had taken more vitamins, what if I had exercised a lot, what if I had eaten different, ... What if, What if ?

But there was no way I could turn back time. I realized I just had to get up, get dressed and go to Dr. Pupa's office and hear the rest of the bad news. My husband and I didn't do much talking that morning while we were preparing to leave and on the ride to Meridian to see Dr. Pupa.

We arrived at Dr. Pupa's office and a few minutes later we found ourselves back in the same room we had been in the day before. As we sat there waiting on Dr. Pupa we spoke no words and suddenly I began crying.

About that time the door swung open and it was Dr. Pupa. She took one look at me and said "Oh" and she came running over to my chair and knelt down on her knees and wrapped her arms around me and held me while I cried. I knew, without looking at Bob, that he was sitting there with tears in his eyes too. I am sure he felt helpless. Dr. Pupa was so precious to me. I have always said that if anyone other than Dr. Pupa had told me that I had cancer I don't think I would have been able to take it. She is definitely "God Sent".

Once Dr. Pupa stood up from holding me in her arms, I began to ramble in my words. I was saying, "I don't want to be here." I put my hands over my ears and said, "I don't want to hear what you have to say, but I need to hear what you have to say". I told her to go ahead and give me the bad news, and to tell me what kind of cancer I had. She said, "I have already told you." I said, "What?" She said, "invasive and non-invasive ductal carcinoma". I said, "Oh, I thought you were going to tell me that I had hodgkins lymphoma or some long, terrible name like that."

I was a basket case, let me tell you. I then went on to tell Dr. Pupa that it was probably spread all over my body. She said, "we don't know that!" I then said, "well, you said it is rare to be in both breasts like this." She said, "it is rare but we have seen it". I said, "well, it is probably fast acting." She said, "we don't know that!". I asked her if she had seen any other cases this bad and she said "I have seen worse". She really had all of the right answers for me at that time. She went on to tell me that I was getting way ahead of myself and that I needed to take this one step at a time and not look too far ahead….That was such good advice and I have been trying to follow it since that day.

We went ahead with the appointment then and she asked me which surgeon I wanted for my mastectomy. I had spoken to a dear friend the night before and she recommended Dr. William Billups, III. I am so glad she did, he is wonderful.

Dr. Pupa then scheduled me for an appointment with Dr. Billups for the following Monday in order that I could schedule the radical mastectomy. The thought of having cancer was bad enough but now my mind shifted to the fact that I would have to have both of my breasts surgically removed. It hadn't been too many months ago that I had told my husband I didn't know how women coped with having breast cancer and losing their breasts and hair, and that I hoped I would never have to deal with that. Now I would have to wait three more days to see the surgeon. This would definitely be a LONG weekend..

I told Dr. Pupa thanks and bye and I told her that I would keep in touch with her on how I was doing. She said that she would like for me to do that because so many times she loses touch with patients and never knows how they did. We have stayed in touch with each other and I am thankful for my new friend.

I am a firm believer that God brings certain people into our lives for a reason. I also believe there are angels among us. Both of these statements are true as it relates to Dr. Sandra Pupa. An Angel that was sent into my life by God for a reason.

Chapter VIII
"Friends and Family Rally Around Me As Support"

A friend loveth at all times, and a brother is born for adversity.

(Proverbs 17:17)

I was amazed at the outpouring of support for me from the very beginning of my journey with cancer.

I looked forward to the mail running every day because I would get a hand full of cards from friends and family to let me know they were thinking about me and praying for me every day. That is such a reassurance to know that people care and are praying for you. A person can never receive too many prayers, especially when they are going through a trial like "cancer".

Since I had retired from East Mississippi State Hospital almost ten years earlier I had lost contact with a lot of my friends there. When you aren't working in the public and you aren't out and about a lot you wonder sometimes if you have any friends anymore. Then you experience a catastrophic illness like I have and you find out that you really do have a lot of friends and support out there.

I kept a basket handy in my den and every time I would get a card in the mail I would read it and then put it in the basket. For months I would get many cards a day and I still receive cards all along. They are so uplifting and they keep me focused on getting well. It does a heart good to know that people do care.

I have always enjoyed sending cards and letters to people but I never really realized how much those cards could mean to someone until I was on the receiving end of it. Thanks to all who thought of me and were so faithful to send me cards and to pray for me. I love you all!

I was diagnosed in October of 2005 and in November, 2005 I received a large package in the mail.

The return address was the "Steel Magnolias and Bear Huggers" from Alabama. I had no idea how they knew about my situation but was so excited to receive the package. It was like an early Christmas. It turns out that they were a "breast cancer support group". Then I found out that my daughter worked with a girl whose mother, Pam, had gone through breast cancer and she lived in Alabama and this was a breast cancer support group that she belonged to and her daughter, Jennifer, had told her about me.

The package contained their news letter, perfume, body lotion, all kinds of little caps and do-rags for me to wear when the time came that my hair fell out. They also had a little bear in there to represent the "bear huggers" and I considered myself hugged at that moment. They had made little pillows, they had a pretty pair of earrings included. It was just a wonderful gift that lifted my spirits, and believe me I needed my spirits lifted. I was crying a lot and still in a bit of shock over the diagnosis. I will never forget how much that package meant to me. I wrote them a thank you note and it was printed in their next newsletter. They had a wonderful poem in there entitled "Steel Magnolias" which talked about the scars across their chest but also their strength. They are still nice enough to mail me their newsletter every month which I enjoy reading very much. Thank you very much Pam and the other ladies in this group of supporters.

It wasn't very long then that my friend Jackie, that I had worked with for almost thirty years at East Miss. State Hospital, called me and said that she had a basket of goodies from my friends at the hospital. She brought the basket to me and it had so many nice things in there. There were cards, candles, body lotions, slippers, plaques with messages like "prayer changes things", "have faith" and "all things are possible", oil lamp, blankets to keep me warm through chemo, bath gels, etc. Again it was like Christmas.

Jackie had included a picture that had been made at work years ago (when we were much younger). It was made on a day we were dressed up for "western day" and we had on our cowgirl hats. She had framed it in a frame that said "Awesome Friends Forever and Always". She has called me and checked on me faithfully throughout this journey. I love you Jackie, very much and I love all of you that contributed to my basket of joy……..

My cousin, Lillian was constantly sending me cards and gifts through the mail. She and her husband, Bill have encouraged me all the way through this. They would not let me get down or let me give up.

I would love to name each and every one that brought me a gift or sent me a card but I wouldn't have room in this book to name each and every one. I just pray that all of you that have thought of me and done for me know just how much you mean to me.

The people that attended the churches where I was going were such a blessing to me always. They encouraged me in my singing and they encouraged me through this trial. They built me up all of the time by telling me I looked good or telling me positive stories about "survivors" of cancer. I will never forget these wonderful people as long as I live.

At one church, Coopers Chapel, there were two women in particular that I knew had gone through breast cancer. I knew about it from the time I had started attending their church. I had always wondered how Peggy and Jewel made it through that terrible disease and all they had to go through like chemo, surgery, losing their hair and being so sick. But I was looking at two victorious women who had come out on the other side of cancer and they both looked "great" and were so energetic and vibrant. One thing that really stood out to me was that both of these women were such "Christian" women. You can just see Christ in them. I wondered if they had always been that way or did they reach that point after experiencing that terrible illness?

I never knew that I would be following in their footsteps and experiencing "breast cancer". I thought of them immediately after being diagnosed and I called both of them to tell them about me.

They were both so sweet and encouraged me so much and tried desperately to give hope to someone that was scared to death that she might be leaving this earth soon. Peggy had gone through breast cancer twice. She had one breast removed and later the cancer returned to the other breast and she had to have it removed and go through chemo just as before. Bless her heart. One time is enough…. But she made it through both times and the cancer has never spread to any other part of her body and it has been twelve years. The doctors are even surprised that it did not spread. It has been over five years since Jewel's cancer and she looks great too and the cancer has not spread. God has been with these two ladies that's for sure.

When you have cancer you look for all of the success stories you can find. I have watched these two ladies and they are an inspiration to me and they give me hope for a future.

I attended Wesley Chapel Methodist Church also and everyone there has been there for me during this trial. Although we have a small congregation, each and every one of them are so loving and kind. I felt right at home the first Sunday I went there. They welcomed me with opened arms. They are special people and mean so much to me. They also encouraged my singing and would never be critical of it because they knew I was trying to serve my Lord. You could tell that they were hurt that I had cancer. They have been with me throughout this trial and I appreciate it very much.

The church I had attended for over twenty years, Hawkins Memorial Methodist Church, has a congregation that is like my family also. It has a small congregation also that is very loving and kind. I decided to start visiting other churches closer to my home back in 2004.

My mother hated to see me leave her church but I wanted to visit around closer to home. I know today that this was in God's plan. I didn't know it then but looking back I know it had to be God's plan. My niece had been singing at our church since she was a child, but I had never had a desire to sing solos. I didn't even like to sing in the congregation because I was afraid someone would hear me. But God knew He wanted me to sing for Him because He knew I was going to have cancer and singing would get me through it. When I began going to Coopers Chapel Methodist I "accidentally" got into singing. You will hear more about that later in this book. The point I am making is that if I had stayed in my comfort zone and stayed at Hawkins church I would never have ventured out and tried singing. Now I love singing. I still do not like my voice but I pray every day that God will give me a beautiful singing voice someday that I will like. I continue to step out on faith and sing for my God...I am so glad I left my comfort zone or I wouldn't be experiencing the wonderful things I am experiencing with my singing today. I do miss the wonderful friends I had at that church and I do visit sometimes but I have a lot of work to do for my Lord and it takes me many places now. Thank you God.

The purpose of this chapter in my book is to tell you what a blessing friends and family are. Another precious gift from God. He provides these friends and family to help get us through our trials.

He speaks to their hearts and prompts them to say and do the right things at the right times. He knows exactly what we are experiencing and knows exactly when to send the right person to give us some gift or some message that we need from God. The friends and family don't even realize a lot of times that they are being used by God to deliver these messages of comfort to us. I try to tell them when they have come at the right time and that God must have sent them. They should be honored that God used them as his tool to deliver messages of comfort. They are blessed too. I want you to know that whatever trial you are in or you are ever faced with that our God will provide exactly what you need when you need it. He is ever present.

Before continuing on to the next chapter I would just like to mention a few other special people that have come into my life during this journey.

I was invited to sing at the Lauderdale County Relay For Life Reception that was held at the Miss. State University Campus in June, 2006. After singing my song, a sweet lady named, Gena, who had introduced me, walked up to the stage and told me that her mother had been through breast cancer and she had made a breast cancer pillow for her and she wanted me to have it...I hugged her and of course it made me cry to think she would think of me in this special way. After the reception was over I went over to thank her and to find out some more about her mother's illness and progress. She told me that she had been diagnosed a couple of years earlier but had actually died from congestive heart failure. She told me that she made the pillow after her mothers death in memory of her. That made the pillow mean even that much more to me. What a precious woman to give up that pillow to me, a lady she had just met. God will bless her for this I know; and I will never forget that day or her as long as I live.

Also, after starting my chemo therapy I was at the Cancer Center one day and noticed a couple sitting across from me. The man was taking chemo and was asleep. He was an older man and a tall and big man, like my daddy. The lady with him, which I assumed was his wife, sat quietly reading a book. After a little while I began talking to her and later he woke up and joined in on the conversation. I found out that he had gone through colon cancer at one time and they cured him. The colon cancer had now metastasized to his liver and he was taking massive doses of chemo. He would come to the cancer center about three days a week and stay for hours taking chemo and then they would fix him up a little machine to take home with him, which administered chemo to him overnight. He seemed to be doing well, considering he was taking so much "poison"…I knew that God had to be taking care of him like He had been taking care of me. I just really enjoyed meeting this couple. His name was Coleman and she was Hilda. As it turned out I was wrong about them being married. His wife was deceased and her husband was deceased and they were friends. She came with him every time he came for treatment. She was a faithful friend. I came to love them both.

I had been asked to write an article for the Meridian Star Newspaper Relay For Life Insert in 2006. I did write my article about my breast cancer and how God was taking care of me and going to heal me. Coleman bought a paper and read the article and told me that he let many people read that article. They lived in Alabama and I would call them and they would call me. We all prayed every night for each other. I wrote him letters to try to encourage him and one day after I had written him a letter I saw him at the cancer center and I asked him if he got my letter. He reached in his shirt pocket (the pocket over his heart) and pulled out the envelope with my letter in it. I almost cried right there in front of that sweet man to think it meant enough to him that he was carrying it with him. Bless his heart.

Well it wasn't too long before they called me and told me that they were going to get married. He was doing well, but still taking chemo. The cat scans had shown the tumors were still there, unchanged, so the Dr. was changing him to a chemo medication that you take by mouth in hopes it would work. They had decided to get married because Hilda wanted to be there all the time and be able to take care of him until the end. She told me, "I am going to take care of him anyway, so we might as well be married so I can be with him all the time". She went on to tell me that she knew, of course, that she could go first, you just never know about those things.

Well, that lovely couple did, in fact, get married. Every time I saw them after that or talked to them on the phone they both told me that they were happier than they had ever been and were living life to the fullest. I was so very happy for them.

Then, just five short months after they were married, Coleman called me and told me that Hilda had died the night before in her sleep. I could not believe this. My heart sank and I just felt so sad for Coleman. I drove to Alabama that afternoon to be with Coleman to try to show him that I cared. All I could think was, "maybe God took Hilda on because He knew she wouldn't be able to handle watching Coleman suffer", and He took her quickly and peacefully so that Coleman did not have to see her suffer. Now what about Coleman? What will happen to him, I thought. One thing I did know for certain was that God would take care of him......

Then I received a call from Coleman that the Dr. said his blood work wasn't looking good and that it looked like the oral medication was not working. He was scheduled for a scan and Dr.'s appointment on the same day I would receive the report from my repeat lung cat scan. I told him that my appointment was an hour and a half later than his so I would come to the cancer center at 12 and sit with him and his family while he waited to see Dr. Keady. I did go and sit with him and his two daughters, his granddaughter and his sister. He went in to see Dr. Keady. I went down to see my Radiation Dr. When I had completed my Dr. visit I went back upstairs to see if Coleman was out of the Dr's. office yet. He came out shortly after I arrived back up there. Honestly he looked so sad, like a little "whooped dog". His daughters had Kleenex in their hands and their eyes were red and I was scared for all of them. I walked over to Coleman and he put his arms around me and said, "I am going to take a break for a while because the chemo isn't working and there is no point in taking it if it isn't working". I hugged him and told him, "yeah, why don't you take a rest. God can take care of you." He said, "He has taken care of me all this time and he will continue to". I love the faith Coleman has. We got on the elevator and I hugged him again and told him that God could do more than chemo anyway, and told him to please call me whenever he wanted to talk. He said, "I'll probably call you tonight." And he did

I left the cancer center that day with a big lump in my throat. So scared I would lose my new found friend. Then I remembered the book by Dodie Osteen, "Healed Of Cancer". I am making Coleman a copy and going to mail it to him because he has metastatic liver cancer and that is exactly what Dodie Osteen had and was completely healed by God without any medical treatments. I want to give Coleman the renewed hope that he needs to get through this victoriously...I know God can heal him and I am expecting a miracle in this sweet mans life. I will continue praying for him and doing all I can to help him through this difficult time in his life. I thank God for bringing Coleman and Hilda into my life.

And last, I would like to tell you that when you have to go to the cancer center as often as you do for treatments when you have cancer, that you meet so many people along the way. I try to talk to a lot of them and tell them my story and try to give them hope. There have been several times during this journey that I would talk to people and get their names so I could put them on my prayer list. I would pray for them. Then one day I would pick up the newspaper and see a familiar name in the obituaries. I would go to my prayer list and sure enough it was one of those people I had talked to some time back. Believe me this puts fear in you every time. You think, they looked good when I saw them last time and now they are gone? Then I have to remember that I must keep my eyes on Jesus, no matter how many are falling around me. Please always remember that. Every situation is unique. God is in control of all situations and He does know best.

Just put your trust in Him to do all that is best for you in your life and in your death. This is not our home, we are only passing through. What we have to look forward to is our beautiful, Heavenly home with Jesus our Lord and Savior. Although we all hate the thought of leaving family and friends here on earth, what a wonderful reunion we will all have with our family and friends that have gone on before us.

And as for Coleman, when the Lord does choose to take him home, he will be again reunited with his Hilda. Their marriage was only five months long before she was taken home to her Lord. But the Lord helped Coleman and Hilda have more happiness and love in that short five months than some couples experience in a lifetime, and some couples never experience it at all. Hilda will be waiting with open arms to meet Coleman. And it is a wonderful thing to know that for all of us - - not only will our family and friends be there to greet us but our wonderful God will be there with open arms to accept us and to tell us "WELL DONE, THOU GOOD AND FAITHFUL SERVANT".......

CHAPTER IX
Preparing For Surgery and Treatment

"Fearfulness and trembling are come upon me, and horror hath overwhelmed me"

Psalm 55:5

Like I said, it was a LONG weekend. After we met with Dr. Pupa Friday morning I called my family physicians office and told them that I had bi-lateral breast cancer and needless to say I was a basket case, and I had not slept the night before and that I needed something for my nerves and to help me sleep. They got the prescriptions ready and we went to pick them up. The Naval Air Station Pharmacy had closed at noon so Bob and I took off up to Columbus Air Force Base Pharmacy. I think it did me good to just be riding rather than going back to the house to just think...

I took the nerve pill that night but never had to take the sleeping pill because the nerve pill alone made me sleepy. I managed to sleep pretty good that weekend. The main problem I had was that upon waking every morning I would get up out of bed and begin crying. I would cry for a while without stopping. It finally came to a point that I wouldn't even be able to get out of the bed before I started crying, I would cry as soon as I awoke. I have never felt so helpless in my life. I was so emotional it was hard to pray. Hard for Cathy to pray? I couldn't believe that. I was such a believer in prayer. Why couldn't I pray? I had thoughts like, "God, why did you let me get cancer? Why did you give me cancer?" I felt like I was being punished by Him. I know now that all of those thoughts were coming from the devil. The devil never rests and he loves to steal our joy and our lives. He had stolen both my joy and my life at this point…I finally came to the realization that God did not give me cancer, the devil did. God did, however, allow the cancer, but for a reason. God knows what He is doing, remember? He had been preparing me for some time for this cancer, I just didn't know it. I'll tell you more later in this book about that…

Monday morning finally arrived and my husband and I were off to Dr. Billups office to get me scheduled for a mastectomy. Usually Bob doesn't go with me to the doctor.

He has always wanted me to go with him and I did, but I never expected him to go with me. I am so glad though that Bob realized that something was probably wrong and went with me to Dr. Pupa's office and now to Dr. Billups office. I needed the support..

We arrived at Dr. Billups office. His nurse, Lisa, got me set up prior to Dr. Billups entering the room. In a few minutes Dr. Billups came in and began examining me. He checked the knot in my breast and then felt under my left arm. There was a knot there too which indicated that the cancer had probably spread to a lymph node. I was already aware of that, but I didn't realize how serious that was at the time. Dr. Billups left the room and made a phone call. He was calling the Anderson Cancer Center and speaking to Dr. Dwight Keady.

Upon Dr. Billups return to the examining room he explained to me that usually the plan would be to schedule me for a radical mastectomy right away but this would not be the plan in my case. He explained that I did have lymph node involvement and that meant he was going to have to "save my life first". I will never forget those words as long as I live. I sat there without moving. I don't think I responded in any way. I just listened. He went on to tell me that "what is in your breasts will not kill you, but what gets out into your body through that lymph node will". Well, I wanted to scream right then and tell everybody to hurry up and get this cancer out of me. I was literally scared to death. I had known of so many cases where the breast cancer was found very early, and they only had one little tumor and the cancer still spread and killed them. I knew I was in a really bad situation.

Dr. Billups went on explaining that he had talked to Dr. Keady at the Cancer Center and I would have to start strong chemo right away and the surgery would come later.

What? I would have to walk around with these cancerous breasts on my chests? I wanted them off NOW. Isn't it strange how your feelings change? Just a few months ago I didn't think I could live without my breasts, now all I wanted was to have them cut off. My life was what I wanted to keep now. But I had to take one step at a time just like Dr. Pupa had advised.

You could tell that Dr. Billups and his nurse, Lisa were concerned and felt bad for me. They were very compassionate and I appreciated that. I held up good and didn't cry in his office, that day. Dr. Billups said that I should be back to his surgery center the following morning and he would insert a medi-port into my chest for the purpose of taking chemo. All of this was new to me. The nurse showed me the medi-port so that I would know what it looked like. I don't know why, but I never even realized that inserting a medi-port is considered surgery. I was out of it, wasn't I?

We returned home and that night was hard again. I think by now it had taken its toll on Bob. He was emotional. I decided that I would go to the surgery center with my mother. Mother wouldn't take anything for being there for me. We drove to the surgery center in her car and I left my car at her house. Remember now that she is eighty-eight years old. She has always been so active but in the last few years I can see her going down. I know that for a long time now she thinks that Karen and I just don't care about her or that she is getting old; but I told Karen one time that it is almost like we think if we ignore the fact that mom is getting older and more feeble that she will live forever. I told mom that once too. A lot of times I let mom do things on her own and I probably should have helped her but I just couldn't bear to admit that she is aging and could soon be leaving us.

The night before I was to go to the surgery center I had spoken to special family, Johnnie, Letha and Tammy. I have been so close to them and loved them for years.

About three years ago there was a terrible workplace shooting at Lockheed. Tammy had been my little rice girl in my wedding and now she was all grown up with two children of her own.

Her precious, Christian husband was at work that day at Lockheed when the shooting took place and he was the first one shot and killed. It hurt me so bad to see Tammy and her family have to go through this terrible trial. They are all very Christian people and yes, God carried them through this great loss. Some things we still just do not understand. Why do things like this happen? What was the purpose? What good came out of it? As my daddy always said, "we will understand it better by, and by". (When we get to Heaven)

Anyway, Letha and Tammy were sorry to hear about my cancer and they wanted to see me. We made a lunch date for Tuesday after my medi-port was put in. Like I said, I didn't realize it was surgery. So once mom and I got to the surgery center and I was waiting for Dr. Billups I realized it was getting late. Dr. Billups had an emergency at the hospital and was running late that day. So I asked the nurses to call Letha and Tammy and tell them I was running late. Looking back this is so funny. When I woke up from surgery I got ready to go and came out in the waiting room and Letha and Tammy were visiting with my mom and waiting to take me to lunch. Now the nurses had given me post-op instructions but I didn't realize it. It said not to drive, and to eat jello or something light. Well, I took off with these ladies and we went to Ryans Steak House for a buffet, no less. Then they took me to moms and I got in my vehicle and ran errands. Oh well, you know I think I did better because I did eat a big lunch and drove all around. That's a hoot... And I thank Letha and Tammy for treating me to lunch that day - I had a ball and I needed to relax and have a little fun...

Now that my port was installed it would be time to start chemotherapy the very next day. I had heard the terrible stories about that stuff. Yes, it may save your life, but it has such bad side effects and could it kill me it was such bad stuff? Well, there was nothing else I could do so I prepared for the first treatment.

I told Bob that there was no point in him going with me for chemo. I don't like for someone to have to wait on me and I was sure it would take a while.

My niece, Lori worked at the Cancer Center and that made it nice to see a familiar face the first time I went. I get to see her every time I go for chemo. She is like a daughter to me and I love her and her brother, Johnny very much.

I met with Dr. Dwight Keady that day and he explained to me the plan of action. Dr. Keady is so sweet to me. He takes his time and lets me ask questions, cry, or whatever. He is very understanding and I am so glad that my friend recommended him to me. He said that I would take four strong chemos, one every three or four weeks and then the surgery, then four more chemos, then probably radiation. I asked him wouldn't the radiation hurt my new breasts?, because I thought I was having reconstruction at the same time as the surgery. He explained that I wouldn't have reconstruction for at least six months after surgery so that I wouldn't have problems with infection. I began to cry. My friend, Diane, had her reconstruction surgery at the same time she had her mastectomy, so I thought I was going to do the same thing. Since then though, I have found out that it was really hard on Diane to do it that way. God worked this out for me so that I couldn't have it done that way. I'll be glad to wait..

I then met Dr. Keady's nurse, Stephanie. I love her. She has been so encouraging and sweet to me. She never hurts me when she puts the needle in the port. It is amazing to watch Stephanie work. How do they learn all that stuff? There are needles, tubes, all different steps to giving the chemo.

They give you steroids, nausea medicine, all kinds of things even before the chemo itself. I call the chemo "big red" because it is….Stephanie invited me to give my testimony and sing at her church and I did. I loved it. I always love singing for my lord and telling everyone what he has done for me.

The girls that work with my niece in the cancer center went together and bought some beautiful material for a quilt. It has the breast cancer symbols all over one side of it. (pink ribbons) When you turn the quilt over it is yellow and in big pink letters it says "Aunt Cathy". The girl that made it tied the two pieces of material together with little ribbons all of the way around and they have the breast cancer symbols on them too. They presented me with that and of course, I cried. How sweet of them to think of me in that special way. I know part of the reason they did it too is because they love my niece, Lori and they knew she loved me and they wanted to do to this for me. I laugh now and say that I inherited 25 more nieces at the cancer center.. Thanks to those sweet girls…

Everyone at the Cancer Center is so sweet and it sure does make it easier to go there for treatments.

After the first treatment I went home waiting for all of the bad side effects. I was already in so much pain. I was hurting all in my back and my ribs. I was sure that the cancer was spread all over my body. My body scan wouldn't be for another week. I believe there was a reason for that too. God worked that out so that I could be anointed with oil and prayed for before the scan. He knows what he is doing, remember?

I had so many people praying for me. Churches everywhere were praying. People had me on prayer lists on the Internet even. Thank God for prayers!

I had been through my first chemo by now. I had asked the nurse if there was a chemo that didn't make your hair come out. She told me "not for breast cancer". Stephanie went on to tell me that my hair would come out in ten days. "A little over a week and I would be bald,"I thought. I went home from chemo wondering how I was going to feel. Would I be sick? She had put nausea medicine in my drip and also had given me a prescription for nausea pills. I had heard about people losing so much weight because they were so sick. I dreaded that most of all. I prayed so hard to God to not let me be sick and to somehow make it through this chemo without a lot of complications. God is faithful………

About two days after chemo I became really weak. Now I had thrown my hormones in the garbage because I saw an ad just before I first went to the doctor, and the ad had said that some hormones can feed cancer. Thinking I might have cancer I had stopped taking them immediately. Now my breasts hurt so bad I couldn't touch them. Of course, I thought all the pain was from the cancer. I was so weak that I didn't feel like getting up out of my chair. I slept a lot and felt hot one minute and cold the next. I was miserable to say the least. Finally I thought, "if I could only get out of this recliner and get to my music room I would try to sing". I drug myself back to the music room and put a CD in.

Now I told you earlier in this book that God knows what He is doing. He knows what is going on in your life and mine. He knows what is going to happen in our life. I am a firm believer that God knew that I was going to have cancer and He knew that singing would help me get through the cancer.

I had left my mothers church and started visiting a church closer to my home. The church was Coopers Chapel Methodist Church in Quitman, Ms. I had started going there about two years prior to my cancer diagnosis. One night a month several people from the church would visit the Lakeside Nursing Home in Quitman and sing for the residents there. They invited me to go and I would play half of the songs on the piano and the regular pianist, Diane, would play the other half of the songs.

One night the leader of the group, Horace, came over to me and asked me if I would do a special. I thought he meant to play a special on the piano. He and his wife and several other people would bring CD's and sing solos, duets, etc. Now I have never sang a solo or duet and I would never even sing in the congregation for fear someone might hear my voice. Well, when Horace asked me to do a special he walked off to continue the song service and I thumbed through the hymn book looking for a song to play on the piano. In a few minutes Horace stood up in front of everyone and said, "Now Mrs. Cathy Riley is going to come and sing for us." I said really quick, "Oh, I don't sing". He laughed and said, "well ya'll need to tell me these things." Everyone laughed and we went on with the singing service for the residents.

I felt really bad that night that I may have embarrassed Horace or hurt his feelings, which I would never want to do. I thought about it a lot. I guess God was working on me and trying to convince me to sing. My niece, Lori, had always sang at my mothers church. I loved to hear her sing. She had a beautiful voice and I never once thought about singing. I hated my voice. But you know God has a sense of humor and he wouldn't leave me alone about it. He knew that He could work on my emotional side and make me feel bad about "letting Horace down". God does know what He is doing, remember?

Well, I went and bought me a karoke machine and my cousins, Lillian and Bill gave me a bunch of cassette tapes that you can sing with. I began practicing. Still I hated my voice. I kept asking God why He wanted me to sing, when I don't have a good singing voice. He still wouldn't let up on me though. Before long I went to Corinth, Miss. To visit my cousins, Bill and Lillian. We sang and they let me sing. When I left up there I decided that I was going to sing at Coopers Chapel the next Sunday. Let me go back for a minute. I had attempted to sing a song a few weeks prior to this at a ladies meeting at the church. I had a very weak and soft voice and I thought they would have a microphone there, but they didn't.

Needless to say I know that the ladies couldn't even hear my voice that day. They were sitting right in front of me but I could tell they couldn't hear me, but they listened and clapped when I was through singing. I was so glad when that song ended and I could sit down. I was so embarrassed. Those ladies were so sweet to me and encouraged me and would have never hurt my feelings for anything. I appreciate their tolerance of my singing. I love every one of them.....

Well, like I said I went to Corinth and sang with my cousins. They were coaching me. Good coaches! When I came home to Quitman I was fired up and wanting to try to sing at church on Sunday morning. I really couldn't believe I was going to try that. That church would be full of people. Did I dare? But God wanted me to I felt like, so I was determined to try.

I went to Coopers Chapel that Sunday morning with confidence that Lillian and Bill had instilled in me. When the time came to sing I walked up to the pulpit, made a little talk and told them I didn't have a singing voice but I was going to sing for my Lord. I sang "Master of the Sea" and I did better this time because I had a microphone. Well, at least they could hear me this time, but I still hated my voice and they just tolerated it. I kept questioning God, "Why do you want me to sing? This is ridiculous. But my God knew what was ahead for me...

So, like I was telling you earlier, I'm weak from my first chemo and I want to sing for my Lord. Somehow I made it to my music room and put a CD in. I began singing with my microphone and the more I sang the stronger I became. I was convinced that day that God had been preparing me for two years for this cancer and treatments. He knew that I would love trying to sing and that it would give me strength to get through the chemo. It has worked every time. I was so weak from chemo one Sunday night that I could barely walk down the church aisle to my pew. It was a fifth Sunday night singing service and they had asked if I wanted to sing. Everyone that sang that night were singing two or three songs and someone asked me to.

I said, "I've had chemo and I'm so weak that I'll do good to sing one song". I went up to the pulpit and sang a song, "I Can't Even Walk Without You Holding My Hand". I went back to my seat. When I walked up to the pulpit I felt like I could barely walk and felt like I was staggering. I made it up there though and made it through the song. Once I returned to my seat I felt so strong that I asked Louise, the preachers wife if I could sing another one. She motioned for her husband, Gerald, the preacher, and he came over and I asked him if I could sing another one. He said, "sure". I had to go to the car and get another CD. They introduced me again and this time I literally bounced up to the pulpit. I asked the congregation if they could see what God can do? I told them that I had been so weak when I arrived at the church that I could barely walk down the aisle. I explained to them that the singing was making me strong and that God had strengthened me on that first song I had sung and I was ready to sing another one. They were clapping and praising God. Do you see how God prepares us for things that we will have to experience? He knew that if I would start singing for Him that the singing would strengthen me and get me through this terrible disease. I thank God every day that He called me to sing, although, I still do not like my singing voice. I am praying that He will give me a better singing voice...

I am so thankful that all of the prayers that went up for me about this cancer and the treatments were answered by our God. I did have four or five days of weakness because the chemo not only kills the cancer cells but also your good cells and brings your body and your immune system down to nothing. However, God did answer many prayers about the nausea. I never had to take any nausea pills. I was told not to get around sick people because I wouldn't have any resistance and I would get sick. I can't tell you how many sick people I did get around and I never caught anything. My God had built a hedge around me and I was protected...The only side effect that I did have was that I lost all of my hair. I never dreamed I could go through cancer, losing my hair or my breasts, but my God was ready, willing and able to go the distance with me to get me through this. He does not put more on us than we can bear!

CHAPTER X
"Clinging To My God and God's Word"

"The grass witherith, the flower fadeth: but the word of our God shall stand forever"

Isaiah 40:8

All I could do was cry upon waking up every morning now. At first I would get up in the morning and begin crying, then it came to a point that I would begin crying as soon as I awoke - before I could get out of the bed.

My ribs were hurting so bad in the front and the back of my body. I just knew I was ate up with cancer all over my body. I had not had my body scan yet. I had begun chemo on November 2nd and my body scan would not be done until November 9th. That was a terrible week of thinking the cancer was in my bones. When Wednesday, November 9th came I went to the hospital and was escorted to a mobile unit in the parking lot. The technician put a needle in my arm to administer the dye. I began crying. I explained to him and the other technician that he had not hurt me with the needle, I was just so worried because I had been diagnosed with bi-lateral breast cancer and I was afraid it was spread over my body. He was so nice. They both were. They brought me Kleenex and you could tell they hated to hear that I had cancer.

Once the time had passed that I had to wait for the dye to travel through my body, they showed me to a room with a bed there. The bed would move and carry you through the tunnel like machine that would make the pictures. I asked both of those technicians to please pray that the cancer would not show up in my body. They said they would pray and I believe with all of my heart that they did pray for me.

As I lay in that really white room, all alone, I prayed.

My prayer was, "Dear Lord, please touch me with your healing hand. Please make all of these tests show that I do not have cancer anywhere other than my breasts." As I lay there I looked toward the white wall to my right and I visualized Jesus standing there with his long hair, beard, white robe and sandals. He was so real to me. I then turned my head so that I was looking straight up at the ceiling. I closed my eyes and I visualized Jesus taking his nail-scarred hands and laying them on my head with that healing touch. I really believed that if I did have cancer anywhere else that He was taking it away right then.

My husband and I left the hospital soon. That night I was scheduled to give my testimony and sing at Christian Fellowship Church in Meridian. The preacher, Sephus, had gone to school with my brother Richard who had died in 1985, and my mother would visit his church some. That afternoon I received a call from Vince, my former boss at East Miss., and he said that he had been going to that church some and had been told I was coming that night to sing. I told him yes. He had been checking on me since the time I had told him about my cancer. He is a very caring person and very unselfish.

That night mother and I arrived at the church and Vince was there. I had friends from mothers church there too, Norma and Louise. I did get up and tell everyone about my cancer and that I had the body scan that day. I was in a lot of pain that night and scared to death I might be going to die. I sang "Master of the Sea". As soon as I finished singing the preacher, Sephus, ran up to the pulpit with tears in his eyes and asked if he could pray with me. I was thrilled. I stepped down in front of the pulpit and he and four other preachers came up and he anointed me with oil and they all prayed for me. There is so much power in being anointed with oil and having them pray for you. I was at peace during those prayers.

At the end of the service everyone of us in the congregation came to the front of the church and had prayer. I was still hurting so bad. I would have to wait until the next day to find out the results of the body scan. But I knew in my heart that even if the cancer had spread to my bones all of these prayers were going to take care of it.

I would pray every time I woke up that night.

The next morning I was going to the grocery store and had just gotten into the car at my mothers house to leave. My cell phone rang and it was Stephanie, Dr. Keady's nurse. She said that Dr. Keady said to tell me that he didn't see any "hot spots" anywhere that he hadn't expected to see them. I asked if that meant that there was no cancer in my bones, liver, lungs or brain. She said yes that was what it meant. I told her everyone's prayers had been answered. She said, "tell them not to stop praying, we are just getting started".

I jumped out of the car and met my mother at the door. I ran into her house and began screaming and crying - poor thing probably thought I had lost my mind. I finally blurted out that I didn't have cancer anywhere else. I ran back to her den and sat down in the recliner and was sobbing. She came in there and put her arms around me, crying too, and we celebrated. Maybe I was going to live after all?

And guess what. After I received the report that all was clear in my brain and the rest of my body all of my pain in the ribs went away. Now that makes me believe that all of that pain was from the devil. He had been working on me since the first day I was diagnosed. He would say, "You waited too long to go to the Dr.", "It's too late", "You are going to die". Now I believe he had put this pain in me to scare me even more but now that the reports proved to be negative and I knew it he gave up on that approach. He is ever present and wants to steal our joy and our life. Don't let him....

Well there was a spark of hope for me now. At least it wasn't spread yet. Now I would try to take a day at a time, again...Stephanie had told me my hair would be out in 10 days. Well I was approaching ten days now and no sign of my hair going. I thought that maybe God was going to let me keep my hair. I surely did hope so.

On the fifteenth day since my first chemo I woke up that morning and went in to brush my teeth. Then I began brushing my hair and this huge lump of hair came out in my brush. Oh no, it is happening. This went on a few days. My hair was getting flatter and flatter. You could not see my scalp because I always had such thick hair that it really was just thinning out. I didn't look like me though because my hair wasn't full anymore. My husband and I drove to the mall and I went to the wig shop. I had always thought I wanted to try a wig but never had. Now I would HAVE to wear one. I went in and it was harder to find one my length and color. I finally settled for a reddish tint wig that was way too long. It was way down on my back which was a lot longer than I was use to, but I bought it. Nothing else would do that they had. When I got back in the car with my husband I just began sobbing. Bob is use to the tears by now but he wondered why I was crying now. I told him I just didn't want to go through losing my hair and having to wear a wig.

I got home with the wig and I hated it. I called my daughter and told her I hated it. I called Sherrill, my best friend from Jr. High and High School. She was a beautician and I asked her if she could trim the wig to make it more my length. She was so nice and told me I could come over the next day. I went to her shop and she loved the wig. I still didn't. She put it on my head and cut it to my length. I liked it better. She wouldn't take a dime for cutting it but she held me in her arms while I cried. She knew I was distraught and she had tears in her eyes too. I know that the day I called and told her that I had cancer she began praying right there on the phone with me. She did not want her close friend to have to go through any of this either.

She is a good friend and I love her dearly. She has prayed often on the phone with me. It is a wonderful thing when you ask someone to pray for you and they begin praying right then and right there..Then you don't have to wonder if they are going to really pray for you.

Now the weekend was approaching and I was suppose to go to Florida and pick my grandson up and bring him to Mississippi. Thank God the chemo side effects didn't last but a few days and I was ready to travel. God always gave me strength to keep traveling to get Cody, even though many people had told my husband and I that once I stayed on chemo a while I would probably not be able to be traveling. I am so glad God blessed me in this way too.

I told my husband that I didn't want to wear my wig to Florida and just walk up for Karen and Cody to be shocked by it. As I said, my scalp was not showing yet, my hair was just thin. So I carried the wig with me, along with my do-rags, caps, etc. When I went by to see my daughter at work I walked in and she was standing across the room. The look on her face showed her sadness, even though she was trying to be strong and smile at me. I really looked like I had been standing out in the rain and my hair had flattened to my head. She told me later that it was obvious I had lost hair even though there were no bald spots. She was used to my full hair.

While there I put the wig on and modeled it for Karen and Cody. Karen really bragged on the wig and did everything she could to make me feel good about it. I still hated it but didn't say anymore about it.

When I took Cody back to Florida at the end of the weekend I spent the night and my hair was really coming out now. I had heard about so many women waking up and finding all of this hair on the pillow or in the bed or all over their house, but mine didn't do like that. It came out by the hands full when I would brush my hair. Then I told my daughter one day that I was beginning to look like the crypt keeper. She laughed and I did too. She hadn't seen my head in a few days. I told her I wanted to show her. I told her to brace herself. We were standing in her apartment at the bar and I took the do-rag off of my head. By now I had a patch of hair here and a patch of hair there. She smiled that forced smile again and said, "that's sort of what I expected". I knew she wanted to burst into tears but she managed not to. I love her so much and it hurt me to know she was hurting for me. We then went to Cody's bedroom to show him. He sat there a minute and looked at me but being the sweet little boy he is he didn't let on that it bothered him. As a matter of fact he told me I looked like another lady we knew, and we got a big laugh out of that. I'm afraid that wouldn't have been a compliment to her but you know a child's honesty....

That night when Karen and Cody were sleeping I slipped into Cody's bathroom, razor in hand and I shaved my whole head. I liked it better like that. My grandson saw it the next day and he absolutely loved it. He loved to take my do-rag off and rub my head. He told me one night that he didn't want me to grow my hair back because he loved the way it felt bald. Now, I loved Cody so much and would do anything for him, EXCEPT that. I wanted my hair to come back just as soon as it could come back; but it would be a while yet.

I would like to tell you though that I have never missed my hair. God took care of that and it is amazing how everything changes when you know that you have cancer. Things that use to mean everything to you mean nothing to you now. My life - and living to see Cody grown was my main goal now.

So I made it through the "losing the hair" ordeal thanks to my God. I had made it through the body scan victoriously too thanks to God, and I was making it through the chemo pretty well too, thanks to God. He is awesome and I was beginning to realize just how awesome.

I was trying to keep my focus on God and His word. I realized that Cody had become the center of my life for the past nine years. I loved him so much and had always told him, "I love you more than life". Be careful what comes out of your mouth...I realized now that I had to rearrange my priorities. I had to put God first in my life and Cody second.

I had always loved my God and I had been singing regularly in churches for two years and was loving that; but when you get a cancer diagnosis and you think your life is over you really look at your life and want to do everything you can to live for your God for whatever time you have left. I think that the devil gave me cancer because I was singing for my Lord and going to church regularly. Now it was time to show that devil that even though he gave me cancer I was still counting on my God and going to live for Him not the devil. That is just what I began doing.

It is amazing too how many well-meaning people will make negative comments about cancer when you tell them you have cancer. This didn't happen too much to me but a few. I knew that the devil was at work in that trying to discourage me. I heard horror stories of people that didn't make it or how bad they suffered. I didn't need any negativity only positive statements. Do not let anyone make negative statements to you. If they begin to tell you something negative just stop them and explain that you are trying to stay positive and you need only positive feedback. They will understand - and if they don't well that's okay too. Just protect yourself from the devil.

Now that I was reading my bible so much and experiencing what God was doing for me through this journey with cancer I wanted to tell everyone I saw. I began not only singing at the churches I attended but I also began witnessing and telling people what God was doing for me. I was trying to give hope to everyone in case they were faced with trials, which everyone will be at some time or another.

I was loving every minute of this testifying. I felt God with me all of the time. He had drawn nearer to me than I could have ever imagined. God is waiting for us to depend on Him. He wants us to call on Him for help. Remember that.

CHAPTER XI

"Every Day There Was Evidence Of God's Presence"

"And I heard a great voice out of heaven saying, behold, the tabernacle of God is with men and He will dwell with them, and they shall be His people, and God himself shall be with them, and be their God."

Revelation 21:3

After a week and a half had passed of crying, worrying, going through chemo and finding out that it hadn't spread yet I was beginning to talk with God and tell Him that I was in a battle and I could not handle this battle alone. He knew my fear and my sadness. He felt the urgency in my prayer, I'm sure. I decided right then and there to let God take over and handle this battle. I could not. From that day forward I had such a peace come over me that it was so good to know He would handle it.

When I returned to Dr. Keady four weeks later for another chemo I asked him if I could see my body scan report. He handed me a green sheet of paper and I began reading the report. A lot of it was mumbo jumbo to me. I don't know all that medical talk. However, I did pick up on the part that said "this patient has a mass in her liver and we recommend further testing" and something about my bones and they recommended further bone scans. My heart sank and I handed the report back to Dr. Keady and asked him, "What does that mean about my bones and liver?" He explained again that when you do body scans there are "hot spots" that show up if cancer is in an area and he had NOT seen those hot spots in my bones or liver or anywhere other than my breast. I trusted him but I was still so afraid. I had been hurting in my right side in about the location of your liver. Did I have cancer in my liver now?

My God knew my fear and concern. The following days were my bad days on chemo with a lot of weakness, sweating, etc. You do feel like you are dying sometimes during chemo.

Your body is just down to nothing. Always on the Sunday after chemo I would go to church, because I knew the devil didn't want me to, but I was always crying on those Sundays because my body was down to zero. All of my friends at church understood that I was crying because I felt so bad from the chemo and couldn't help the tears. They were so understanding. Well this particular Sunday I went to Wesley Chapel Methodist Church and walked in and was crying. They would always hug me and pray for me. What a blessing they all were and are. I had not discussed with anyone there about my concern over the body scan report and my liver.

God is an all-knowing God. God uses people to comfort us. He prompts people to call people at certain times, to pray for them or give them things, etc. Little did I know that God was going to comfort me that very morning and take my latest fears away. When I went into the sanctuary after the hugs from my friends, I was standing and talking to a lady named Lucy. Another lady, Louise, walked up to me and didn't say anything to me, she just had a little green book that she laid on top of the bible in my hands. I didn't really notice at the time what it was. After church I looked at it and the title was "Healed of Cancer". I went to her and asked if she had given me the book and she said "yes". I thanked her, not knowing what a great blessing and comfort that little green book would be to me.

After lunch that day I sat down and read that little green book. It was written by Mrs. Dodie Osteen, Rev. Joel Osteen's mother. It told all about her being diagnosed with metastatic LIVER cancer and the doctors sent her home with no chemo or treatment of any kind and told her she had three weeks to live. It told about how she got in God's word and prayed all of the time. It told how she found God's promises about healing and she had about forty plus scriptures that she read every single day. Yes, she suffered and felt like she was going to die many times.

She and her husband prayed, prayed and prayed. The little book also told me that "God is the same yesterday, today and forever". It made this statement many times throughout the book and even the last line in that book was that statement. My preacher, Pam, delivered the sermon that day and it was "God is the same yesterday, today and forever". Now, can you see how God works?

He was the only one at that church that day that knew I was worried about my LIVER. So He chose Louise to bring me that little green book that not only discussed Dodie Osteens liver cancer but it told me that she was completely healed and was still alive 26 years later. Hers was a hopeless situation, so the doctors thought, but God healed her because of her faith. He also used my preacher that day to bring me a message of hope that God healed yesterday he can heal today and forever. My God orchestrated that whole Sunday morning service for ME that day. Praise God how I love Him…

I found out that day also that Louise had cancer years ago. Her husband, Jimmy, came up to me after church and told me that she had one of the worst cancers, I think a type of bone cancer, over twenty years ago and she had been healed. She was fine today. Another story of victory over cancer - another uplifting of my spirit. Thanks.

My fear over my liver left me that day and has never returned. I began reading that little green book every day and reading all of the same scriptures that Dodie Osteen read every day. It has been a great help to me.

There was another couple in that church that had cancer touch their lives. Harold and Nancy were a couple I met when I first started going to Wesley Chapel. I thought they were so nice and friendly but I had no idea that she had been through thyroid cancer about six years earlier. She was so pretty and energetic. No obvious adverse affects of this disease as far as I could tell. I never knew she had been through cancer until I found out I had cancer.

She told me about her cancer, surgery, radiation and that all tests were proving to be normal now. Praise God. Another success story and she looks great. I can hang on to her story to help me get through too.

I had an experience one night where I was in the bed and I began praying. My grandson had called and was crying and worried about me. He said he felt like he needed to be spending time with me. He thought I was going to die, I know. I went to bed and something came to my mind. I began moving my hand in the air and making a circle around my body and praying to God that He would encircle Karen, Cody and I and comfort us and protect us through my illness. I had never thought of that before - asking God to encircle me and my descendants. Where that came from? God.

The very next morning I spoke with my friend, Diane, on the phone and she said she had been reading scriptures that morning and God had led her to type some on the computer.

She began reading those to me. I was standing in a Dollar General Store, of all places, listening to my dear friend read scriptures that God had led her to. I couldn't believe it but she was reading a scripture that talked about God encircling our hearts and the hearts of our descendants. Almost word for word what I had prayed the night before. Every day I was being shown that my God was with me and helping me through friends. What a reassurance.

Then one day I prayed to God that I would love to hear His voice audibly. I had heard of people that had heard His voice, but I never had. A few weeks later I woke up in the night and got out of bed and began praying, "Dear God, please heal me of this cancer, and thank you for everything you do for me." Before I could hardly get the word "me" out of my mouth I heard a man's voice speak up and say "You're Welcome". I turned my head to look in the direction of the voice and no one was there. I knew then that God had answered my prayer and let me hear his voice audibly. I was amazed.

His voice was not loud and booming like you would think it would be and it was not a still, small voice like we have heard He has; but it was just a man's voice like any other man on earth you may know. He did make sure he spoke distinctly though so that I would surely understand what He said. Thank you Lord for speaking to me. I really know now that you are right beside me all of the way and I am in good hands. Thank you for answered prayer again. This further affirmed to me that my God is not only using friends to help and comfort me but He is right here by my side. What a wonderful reassurance that was.

The next night I got up and prayed the same prayer and waited in hopes I would hear His voice again. I didn't. But that is alright. I know He is there whether He ever speaks audibly to me again or not. HE IS HERE.....

Also, there was another couple at Wesley Chapel Methodist Church that had lost one daughter. The lady, Mary, told me that from the first day I attended that church she felt a bond with me. I felt it too. One night she called me and asked me if I was going to have to have a blood transfusion when I had surgery. I hadn't really thought about that yet, but I told her that it would seem that if they were going to cut both of my breasts off that I probably would lose a lot of blood. She went on to tell me that she had taken care of that for me. I asked her what she meant and she said that her daughter, Jeanne, had a type of blood that was compatible with most blood types and that she wanted to donate blood in my name. This was another blessing from God. I couldn't believe that someone I had never met was going to give me her blood (if I should need it). That is a gift of life isn't it? Her daughter did indeed donate the blood in my name for the date of my surgery and to the hospital where I would be having the surgery. She told me that if I didn't have to have blood someone else would benefit from the blood. As it turned out I didn't have to have a blood transfusion but it gave me great comfort to know that someone would benefit from the gift that Jeanne had given for me...Thanks Mary and Jeanne...

Then there was the day I was in Florida and I took my little grandson fishing at the beach on a long pier. There was an elderly man and his son there. They were both professors and we began talking about fishing and my grandson.

I explained to them that I was going to be having a radical mastectomy the next week and I wanted to bring Cody fishing before that. It turned out the elderly man had worked at Oral Roberts University. He asked if I knew of that place. I certainly did and I believe in prayer and healing. I had already asked him and his son to remember me in their prayers and they said they would. But as Cody and I turned to walk away, down the pier, the elderly man called out my name. He said, "Cathy, I would like to pray for you right now." I thanked him and he called his son over there and they prayed for my healing right there on that pier. A pier overlooking a beautiful ocean that our God had created. What a wonderful moment in time that was. Another prayer for healing and a prayer said by a professor that had worked with the healing ministry of Oral Roberts.

God was doing everything He could to let me know He was there, He would help me, He would hear all of these prayers and heal me.

He was telling me also that I needed to build my faith and overcome all of these fears the devil was putting in me.

Finally one day when the devil had just kept on at me trying to put fear in me I had read in the bible that I could rebuke that devil - so I did. I said to the devil "Devil, I rebuke you in the name of Jesus. I have someone much bigger than you on my side so get away from me", and I have never been afraid since. He has left me alone so far..

The devil cannot stand the fact that I am working for my God. He doesn't like me singing or testifying. Guess what? That makes me more determined than ever to serve God. I have told the devil that whatever God has planned for me I will continue to serve Him and that the devil cannot scare me. Even if it is God's plan to take me to heaven I will never turn my back on God and I will not listen to the devil, so the devil might as well go on and leave me alone. I am a child of God now and forever.

CHAPTER XII
"Surgery Date Finally Arrives"

"The righteous cry, and the Lord heareth, and delivered them out of all their troubles."

Psalms 34:17

I continued to go through chemotherapy through the Thanksgiving Season and the Christmas Season. I would have four or five sinking days where I would stay home in my recliner a lot; But God would strengthen me at the end of those few days and I was pretty much back to normal. I enjoyed the holidays as usual. I continued to travel to Florida to get my grandson every other weekend and take him back for school each time.

I was use to my bald head by now. I never wore anything on my head when I was around the house. My husband liked my bald head just like Cody did. I enjoyed going "topless" (no wig) around the house because my head would get so hot in that wig - and it was winter no less. "What in the world would that wig feel like in the summer", I thought. Before long I would be finding out because I would still have to wear a wig in the summer. I remember my pastor, Pam, at Wesley Chapel, hated that I lost my hair, because I was hoping I wouldn't. But Mrs. Anderson, my friend that went to that church, told Pam she was glad that I lost my hair, because to her that meant that the chemo was working. Mrs. Anderson told me about that conversation and further explained to me that her husband had cancer years ago. She said that they gave him chemo and he never lost his hair and he didn't live too long. She felt that the chemo had not worked and she further felt that since I lost my hair that meant that this was a good sign that my chemo was working. I prayed she was right, although I was very sad for her that she lost her husband. They were young when he died and she was left to raise her children all alone. My heart went out to her but I appreciated her sharing this story with me and giving me the hope that my chemo was working and making me feel even better about losing my hair.

I had been through four of the strongest chemos I could take now. February was here.

I visited Dr. Billups III, the surgeon, again and he scheduled my surgery for February 20, 2006. Actually I picked that day. He wasn't too thrilled I don't think, because he was scheduled to go out of town for the rest of the week the day after my surgery. You could tell he didn't like to operate and then go out of town and not be here for his patients. But being the sweet guy he is, he knew the 20th was the best day for my schedule in going to get my grandson, so he went ahead and scheduled it for that day. It would be on a Monday.

I remember I hugged him at the end of the appointment and asked him to "please take good care of me". I choked up thinking about the possibility of not making it through the surgery due to the heart problem I had, which was atrial fibrallation. He promised me that he would take good care of me and I felt relieved at that point. He shook hands with my husband and left the room.

His nurse, Lisa, walked over to the examining table where I was sitting with my hands over my face crying pretty bad. She looked at my husband and said "bless her heart" and she hugged me. She showed so much compassion for me and wanted to comfort me. I appreciated her so much. She began explaining things to me about the upcoming surgery. She told me that Dr. Billups would see patients that morning, February 20th, and then he would leave his office and come on over to the hospital around 11:00 a.m. to do the surgery. I figured he would eat lunch first and then start surgery.

The next step would be for me to go a few days prior to surgery and get pre-registered. I went and they weighed me. I had gained weight because of the chemo/steroids. I hated that part. Then they did a chest x-ray, EKG, and blood tests. The nurse gave me instructions for the day of surgery. I was now ready for the surgery as far as they were concerned; But no, I wasn't ready for surgery as far as I was concerned. Could I go through this?

Was I strong enough? I had heard it was very painful and it would be very painful exercising in order to raise my arms. I remembered just how sick at my stomach I had gotten when I had my hysterectomy years earlier. I was so sick.

My poor mother stayed with me that night of surgery and held my hair back while I vomited. I mentioned this to Dr. Billups and asked if he would give me something so I wouldn't be so sick. He told me that with this type surgery it is inevitable that you will be sick. I dreaded that and the pain so much. I thought, "I'll just have to pray hard about the pain and the sickness, and I'll ask everyone else to pray too, because He has already answered my prayers about chemo, etc. so He can answer these prayers too."

The nurse had told me also that I would probably sleep the rest of that day and maybe into the night, I would be so sedated and on pain killers. I hated the thought of sleeping and missing out on being with my family, especially my daughter and grandson who would only be there Monday and leave sometime Tuesday. Karen has only been back to Mississippi two times since moving to Florida and that was one time when her daddy was shot at Lockheed in one of the worst workplace shootings there had been. Thank God his guardian angels were with him that day and he survived. He was hurt bad. He was shot in the arm and in the back. A lady where he worked put her finger in the hole in his arm to stop the bleeding and held it there until the ambulance came. They said if she had not done that Randy would have bled to death in six minutes. (that was one of two times the guardian angel was with him). The other was that one of the bullets had hit him in the back. The doctor told him that it looked as if the bullet had gone through something or someone before hitting him in the back and when the bullet reached Randy's back it penetrated slightly and fell out onto the ground because it didn't have enough momentum to go on through his back. If it had been going full force it would have gone through his back, through his heart and out the front of his chest and he would have died right there.

We are so thankful that his guardian angels were with him and that God spared his life that day. We are just so sad that so many others lost their lives that day in that shooting. We pray for them and their families.

The second time Karen had come back to Mississippi was when Cody was here visiting us and his daddy. He had gone for a visit to his paternal grandparents house and I received a call from Cody's daddy that Cody had been riding on the back of a four wheeler with his cousin and they had a wreck. It turned out that they were both hurt bad and taken to the hospital. Cody had a broken growth plate in his right leg and it was going to require surgery. As soon as I called Karen she headed to Mississippi to be with him. I know that was a long three hour drive for Karen that night. When you get bad news like that you just want to be there right away, but it doesn't always work out like that. I thank God that Karen got here safely and that God carried Cody through that terrible surgery like He did. Cody did suffer with a lot of pain and it was so hard on all of his family to watch him go through that. His cousin, Victoria, that had been driving the four wheeler went through a terrible time also. It is amazing how God can heal though. You would have thought Victoria would have scars on her face because it looked like she scraped the ground up with her face. But our God healed her completely and I saw her some time back and she is absolutely beautiful. You would never know she had been in that accident. As far as Cody' leg, his surgery scar has lightened up a lot and he runs and plays like nothing has ever happened. However, he does have pins in his leg that will go through life with him and when he falls or bumps that knee it is very painful. I just thank God that he spared the lives of those two children that day.

Anyway, I didn't like the idea of not getting to visit with Karen and Cody the day of my surgery and was hoping I would be able to wake up fairly quick after my mastectomy.

I also thought about my cousin, Lillian, who had driven three hours to get here from North Mississippi to be with me. I wanted to be with her too. I also didn't want to miss any visitors that I might have, if I was going to have any. I figured I wouldn't have much company because they would figure I would be asleep. I love seeing people and I hated to miss seeing anyone. I would pray about the "sleeping" part too.

So my prayer was: "Dear Lord, please help me to wake up soon after surgery. Help me not to have much pain and help me to be able to raise my arms soon without too much pain. I do want to be with my family and friends and visit after surgery. Please help me not to be nauseated after surgery or that night either. I thank you for all of your blessings all my life, but especially throughout this journey with cancer". Amen

I prayed this prayer many times in the days prior to surgery. I was afraid. I had my will updated, and wrote letters to all of my family to tell them how much I loved them. I have told them also that I believe and have faith that God is going to see me through and heal me, but that if he chooses to take me to my heavenly home that I didn't want them to ever lose their faith in God because I died. I told them that if I die from this cancer or during the surgery that God had other plans for me to be with Him and my family that has gone on to the other side. I need for them to always have faith in God like I do. I believe God has plans for ONLY GOOD in our lives and we are all appointed a time to die and we do not know when that is. It is up to God.

I went to Coopers Chapel Methodist Church the Sunday before my surgery on Monday. I told them that I wanted to sing that day because I use my arms to make my motions while I sing and it would probably be a while before I could raise my arms again. Jewel, my friend at Coopers Chapel that had cancer in one breast, had told me on the phone one day that she was going to come to my house and help me with the exercises to get my arms to raise, and that it was going to hurt but I was going to have to do the exercises or I might not ever be able to raise my arms straight up anymore.

I had asked Dr. Billups about the exercises on my last visit and he said they would be giving me some to do after surgery. I knew this was very important so that I wouldn't have a bend in my arm when I raised my arms. I knew of women that even years later couldn't raise their arms straight up because they did not exercise as they should have. I really appreciated the fact that Jewel offered to come and help me like this and I looked forward to her doing just that.

I sang "Calvary's The Reason Why" that day at Coopers Chapel and enjoyed it very much. I was sad to think it may be a while before I could sing and raise my arms like that again. I told the congregation to please pray for me because I was scared and I had never dreaded a surgery so much in my life. I know they did pray as they had always done for me. One of the elderly women of the church, Mrs. Evelyn, we call her, came up to me after church and she said, "I want you do to something. When you go in for surgery tomorrow I want you to "rest in the lord", just rest in the Lord....." I listened to Mrs. Evelyn and decided that I would do just that. That night I prayed and put it all in God's hands. I rested good that night, believe it or not.

Monday morning my husband and I got up and got dressed. I didn't have to get to the hospital until 9:00 A.M. to prepare for surgery. We arrived there on time and went straight to same day surgery.

The nurses and staff there are all very nice. My mother and my cousin Lillian were there when we arrived. Lillian had rounded up a wheel chair to have for my mother because the hospital is so large and mother can't hold out to walk that far.

After I got dressed in that lovely hospital gown and got settled into bed God had moved many of my friends to come to the hospital that day. God knows me and He knows you. He knew that I love people and the best thing for me at that time would be for my friends and family to rally around me before surgery and lift my spirits.

Dalma came from my old church Hawkins Memorial. She is always faithful to visit the sick in the hospitals and she does many, many things for the ladies of the church that need someone to help them get groceries or have errands run for them. She is just in her 90's but she takes care of all the other little ladies. She is remarkable. Then Harvey came in and prayed for me at my bedside. He had attended my daddy's charge in Kemper County all those years ago but he is still a faithful friend to my mother and I. My husband's cousin Cecelia came in carrying a gift from her and my husband's other cousin, Jackie. My pastor at Wesley Chapel, Pam, came in, as I knew she would. She said a pretty prayer at my bedside also.

And to show you that God knows what He is doing. My mother had hired a lady to come and clean her house the week before my surgery. Mother told the lady that was cleaning the house about my breast cancer and my upcoming surgery. The lady, Judy, told mother that her husband worked with another man whose wife had breast cancer in the past and she and Judy were friends. She told mother that this lady, Sylvia, worked as a volunteer with the American Cancer Society. She worked one day a week with a program called "Reach To Recovery"....She promised she would tell Sylvia about me so that maybe she could talk to me. Guess what day Sylvia worked at Andersons? Right, it was Monday - the same day I would be having my radical mastectomy. See how He works things out for those who love Him…

So here I am in my room awaiting surgery and in walks this beautiful, vibrant, energetic red head named Sylvia. She is carrying a bag. She sits down on my bed and introduces herself to me. She begins to tell me her story about her breast cancer. She tells me she had both breasts removed. She tells me she had reconstruction. She tells me that her son was very young when this happened to her and that she was also young. She went on to explain that the doctor had told her that women who are that young when they have breast cancer do not usually live. He gave her a death sentence. But she went on to further explain that her son was now in college and it had been nineteen (19) years since her cancer. She has had no reoccurrence. A truly amazing story told to me by a truly amazing woman. It was a story that I needed desperately to hear that morning. It was a story that gave me reassurance and hope. I looked at her and realized that she had overcome that death sentence and thought to myself, "look at her, she is beautiful. Her hair is gorgeous, she is so full of life and energy. Maybe I can make it through this surgery and this cancer and come out as vibrant and happy as she is." I hope that I can convince Sylvia that she was God sent and that she really played a big part in my doing so well during and after this mutilating surgery. I love her dearly and hope we will stay in contact always.

While she was talking to me my daughter, Karen, arrived from Pensacola. It had been raining that morning and I was worried about her driving her little sports car on the slick roads. That is the mother in me. When she walked through the door I began to cry and she hugged me. Sylvia asked if she needed to leave and let Karen and I have our time together but I said no, because I wanted to know more about Sylvia and her cancer and recovery. I told Karen about what Sylvia had told me so far, hoping Karen would be encouraged also. When Sylvia finished comforting me she gave me a pretty heart-shaped pillow. She said I could use that when driving after surgery. I could put it between the seat belt and my chest to protect me. I did use it for that for a while but since then and until the day of this writing I cuddle it when I sleep. When you have cancer you look for anything you can to bring you comfort and security. As she told me bye she told me that she would be there for me through this and she was and still is.

The next visitors I had were Johnnie, Letha and Tammie. It was so good to see them. Tammie's husband had been shot and killed at Lockheed almost three years earlier. It was one of the worst workplace shootings ever and was the same shooting where Karen's daddy had been shot. Johnnie, Letha and Tammie are family to me too.

They came in my room and visited me. Tammie handed me a little square gift. I opened it up and there was a beautiful, shiny, pink bow shaped pin. I began to cry. I was so overwhelmed by all the friends and family God had sent my way that morning, and the pin was so beautiful and such a sweet gesture from a sweet lady that I had watched grow up. She had been my little rice girl in my wedding all those years ago. Now she is grown with two children of her own. I love her and her family so much. After our little cry we settled down and Johnnie, her dad, asked if he could pray with me. I was thrilled. I called Karen into the room and we all held hands and Johnnie prayed a beautiful prayer. He thanked God for what I had meant to them in their lives - but he didn't know that they are the ones that have meant so very much to me all these years.

My niece, Lori came in to visit and let me know she would be there for the surgery. She told me she loved me and hugged me.

Her husband, Charles, came to see me too. They both know how much I love them and their little girls, Bailey and Lauren.

Then I look up and a man from Wesley Chapel Church, Harold is coming in. I asked where Nancy, his wife, was and he said she should be coming in right behind me. Nancy and Harold have been real nice to me and I had gotten close to them. I was thrilled that they had come to see me before my surgery. However, due to the fact that the doctor was on time, Nancy got there right after they rolled me out of the room. She and Harold did come to see me every day I was in the hospital I think.

I received a call on the phone from Phylis. I was suppose to call and let her know which room I was in when I got settled down, but I hadn't had a dull moment since I arrived. With all the visitors I forgot to call. She found me though and called to wish me luck from she and her husband, Russell. Phylis and their daughter, Michiel had called me on a regular basis since I was diagnosed with cancer. All the visitors and phone calls were truly blessings from God.

All of Karen's daddy's family have been so good to check on me, call me and send me cards. Thanks Judy and Malcolm, Wayne, Esther, Russell, Phylis and Mechiel, Johnnie, Letha and Tammie. Karen's daddy has been good to check on me and help out with Cody too. Thanks to all of you.

My friend, Jackie and her husband, Tommy arrived after I left for surgery too, because I had told them the doctor would probably eat first and be later getting there. They stayed while I had surgery and until they could hear the report from the doctor.

I think I had about fifteen or twenty people that were there before, during and after my surgery. I appreciate it so much and I loved every minute of their visits.

Several of my friends had asked what time the surgery was scheduled for. I told them that the nurse had told me that Dr. Billups would see his office patients that morning and would head over to the hospital about 11 A.M. I knew that so many times doctors are running behind so I told my friends I figured it would be later and that he would probably eat lunch before starting surgery. WRONG…Another wonderful thing about Dr. Billups III is that he was right on time. He showed up at 11 A.M. I think all of my family and friends were amazed by that.

When he showed up I had on my do-rag and my breast cancer cap. He asked, "Are you ready to roll?" I said, "Yes, I have on my cap and I'm ready to roll."

They rolled my bed out into the hall and all my friends and family were there to see me off. I reached my hand out to my precious daughter and said, "come here baby". I was so sad, because I didn't really think I would make it through this surgery for some reason. I was also sad thinking about the fact that sometimes when a mother has breast cancer the daughter will too, and I couldn't stand to think about her ever having to go through it.

She came walking over to me with her pretty little red sweater on, and she leaned down to hug me. I grabbed her around the neck and began to cry and tell her I loved her. I told her twice I know. When I finally let go of her and she stood up I could see the big old tears filling her eyes. She is so precious to me.

At this point I was glad that Cody wasn't there at that moment. We had thought it would be best if he spent the night with Karen's daddy that night and they could come to the hospital later in the day when I got back from surgery. I'm glad he didn't have to see me crying before I went in to surgery.

When I arrived in the surgery area the nurses saw me crying and asked if they had just scared me to death. I said, "No I just had to say goodbye to my baby girl." I had left my breast cancer cap with my husband and now I gave the nurses my do-rag so I could wear the pretty surgical cap they make you wear. That is the last thing I remember before waking from surgery.

When the surgery was over my doctor went to my room to talk to my family. There was at least twenty people (friends) lining the walls by my room. He entered the room and asked who he needed to be talking to and my daughter said "me". He told my daughter that they did find that my right lymph node was enlarged like the left one had been. He said he didn't know if the cancer was spread there or if it was just reacting to the cancer. He further explained that he had done the surgery the old fashioned way because it was spread pretty good in there.

He had scraped my left breast area all of the way up to the collar bone. He also told her that I did have lymph node involvement in the left side for sure and they didn't like to see that. I appreciate his honesty with my family though.

On every surgery I have ever had I remember being taken back to my room and I even remember helping the nurses get me onto the bed in the room. That was not the case in this surgery. I don't remember waking up in the recovery room nor being put into my hospital room bed.

The first thing I remember is hearing my mother saying "he is crying". I knew she was talking about my precious grandson, Cody. I tried desperately to open my eyes. I finally got them to open enough that I turned my head to the right and could see cody in the chair in the corner of my room. His back was turned to me and he had his face against the back of the chair and his little body was shaking because he was sobbing. I couldn't stand to see him crying because I knew he was worried about his "memaw". I put my hand out and told him to come to me. I could feel the oxygen tubes in my nose and knew that he didn't realize what that was and was probably scared. He took my hand, ever so gently, and I told him, "I'm just fine baby, memaw is going to be just fine. I feel great". I understand that earlier he had been crying and my husband, his "papa" had loaned him his handkerchief. Cody loves me and I love him so much.

From that point on I was awake. I realized that I had made it through the surgery and I further realized that I had no pain. I began to realize that every prayer I had prayed that morning was being answered. I had woke up pretty quick after surgery, I had no pain, I hadn't died during surgery, and my friends and family were all around me. People began coming into my room and hugging me. I can't begin to name everyone that came to the hospital but you know who you were and how much I appreciated each and every one of you. They were talking about how bright eyed I was and I was raising my arms and waving at everybody. I was raising my arms. Can you believe it? Another answered prayer.

I began showing everyone how I could raise my arms "straight up" to heaven and I hadn't even been given any exercises to do yet? Thank you God. Several people made the comment later that you could just feel God in that room that day.. I laughed and said don't you know that God had a good time that day. I said that He was probably standing in the corner of the room that day smiling and saying "these people pray and they say they believe that I will answer their prayers, but when I do they are just shocked and amazed."

I do have faith and I do believe God answers prayers but I am still awe-stricken when He answers so many, so fast. Now not all prayers are answered that quickly but He does answer eventually in His time and in His way according to His will. The waiting does teach us patience, doesn't it?

The next day after my surgery my daughter and grandson would be returning to Florida. I did get to visit with them a while and they brought me some beautiful flowers. I love flowers better than anyone probably and believe me I got a room full of flowers and gifts. We ran out of places to put them and began setting them in the floor. I am having a ball at this point. Can you imagine that, after having your breasts cut off. God planned it that way for me.

The night after my surgery, Tuesday night 2/21/06 my husband and I were in the room alone when a doctor came in. He had never met me, didn't know anything about me and that was probably the first time he had seen my medical chart. He told me that there was no cancer found in my right breast and right lymph node. I knew then that God had answered my prayer about showing everyone "Just what He could do" …The cancer had been in my right breast but He healed it. The doctor went on however, to tell me that I had cancer in the left breast with five of nine lymph nodes involved. I asked him what he thought about that and he said, "well you look good, your strong and I think you will fight". I said, "but do women usually live that have that many lymph nodes involved?" He said, "no, it is very difficult, but we will keep you comfortable."

Now I have always said that if a doctor told me that I was dying or had a certain amount of time to live, I would tell him that only God knows when I will die". But I didn't do that. I fell apart. My husband and I both cried. I told the doctor that I was sorry that I was crying and upset. He was holding my hand. He said, "that is alright, that just means you understand what I am telling you". Well

I felt right then and there like I had been given the death sentence, like Sylvia had.

It took me a couple of days to build back up and renew my faith. I discussed it with my cancer doctor, Dr. Keady and he reassured me and reminded me that we knew I had lymph nodes involved from the beginning and that was why we were going to have four more chemos after surgery.

I felt better and back on track. When the doctor returned on Thursday and asked how I was I held my hand up to heaven and said, "I have decided that cancer is a disease from the pit of hell and it is not going to take me out of here. I have faith in my God and He is going to heal me". The doctor smiled and put his hand up and said, "good, give me a high five. Do you want to go home?" and I said , "Yes" and he discharged me that day. Praise God.

CHAPTER XIII
"God Gives Me Strength You Can't Imagine"

"It is God that girdeth me with strength, and maketh my way perfect"

Psalm18:32

As I said, the doctor discharged me from the hospital on a Thursday afternoon. Several ladies at Coopers Chapel Methodist Church had visited me several weeks before my surgery and brought me a basket of gifts from the "care group" at the church. During that visit we discussed the upcoming "Women of Faith Seminar" that would be held at the church on Saturday, February 25, 2006. It sounded wonderful and I knew I wanted to attend really bad. Several people had already told me about it and asked me if I would attend and maybe sing that day. Now these ladies were asking me the same thing. I told them that my surgery was probably going to be on the Monday before that and I didn't know if I would be able to do that or not but I would see.

Well, I'm telling you that God is good and He knew that I loved telling people what He was doing for me. God had blessed me through my strong chemos but this surgery had been a complete miracle with all kinds of prayers being answered. I had such a strong desire to go to this seminar and share with these women my story. I prayed.

Saturday morning, February 25, 2006 arrived. I got out of bed and felt a little weak and nauseated. I prayed for strength to do this. God heard and answered.

Since I was not allowed to drive for two weeks after surgery, my husband drove me to the church. Cars were everywhere. Women had come from all around, Miss., Alabama, etc. I had put a pair of black slacks on and a black slip over top.

Now remember I have forty staples across my chest and four drainage tubes (two in each side). I had taken the drainage tubes with the bulbs on the end that catch the blood, and put them in zip lock bags and pinned them to my top up high on each side. Then I put on a hot pink jacket to hide these tubes. I put on the pretty pink pin Tammie gave me at the hospital. So now I am entering the church looking funny, I know. My jacket flared out on each side, so I looked slim in my legs then fat around my waist area. Oh well, at least I had strength enough to get there.

No one could believe I was able to come, especially me. I am not that strong of a person. It had to be God.

There were over one hundred and sixty women there that day. Most of them I had never seen before because they were from out of town. The seminar started at 8:30 A.M. and lasted until about 4:00 P.M. I stayed all day, thanks to the strength from my God.

There were two ladies assigned to speak that day and several ladies were assigned to sing. One lady was unable to come so I was allowed to sing and give my testimony. It was one of the most wonderful days of my life. Something took me over when I got on that stage. We know who it was, don't we. I began to tell them what I had been through and that I just got home from the hospital two days before and that I had forty staples and four drainage tubes that's why I looked so out of proportion. I opened my jacket and showed them the zip lock bags pinned to my shirt. I told them that Cathy Riley wasn't doing this it was God. He was giving me the strength to talk to them that day and I did. I told them about faith, prayer, believing God for answered prayers and reading the bible and standing on God's promises. They saw with their own eyes what God had done for me and was told what He could do for them as well. That is the purpose of this book also to tell you God is there for you, waiting for you to call on Him and lean on Him. Don't wait. Ask Him anything. He will be there for you...

I pray that someone got a blessing that day from my talk and the two songs that I had the strength to sing. And I had so many women come to me and hug me and tell me I was a blessing to them. But I want everyone reading this to know that no one received a bigger blessing than Cathy Riley did that day. It was wonderful. I got a standing ovation from all of those beautiful women and I just thank God for all He did to help me get there that day and do what I did. All the glory and praise needs to be given to God for that.

I have never felt like I did that day. It was like God took control of me when I got up on the stage of Coopers Chapel Church. When my husband drove me to the church that morning, as soon as we arrived at the church I realized that I had left my notes at home that I had planned to use to speak that day. Well, it turned out that God gave me the words to say and I didn't need any notes. I told my daughter that I felt like Joyce Meyer that morning - I felt like I was preaching and I loved every single minute of it.

Also, up until this day I had not discussed my desire to be a Lay Speaker with anyone other than my immediate family. To show you how God works, while I was giving my testimony that morning God urged me to tell everyone that I was hoping to become a Lay Speaker when I got over my treatments. After I returned to my seat and when the next break came, a pretty woman walked over to where I was sitting and said, "I want to give you this". She handed me a small, folded piece of paper. She laughed and said, "It's not a check" and I said, "I didn't figure you were paying me". (I knew I wasn't that good of a singer - ha) I opened the note and it was her bank deposit slip with her name, address and phone number on it and she had written me a note that read, "Thanks for your faith! When you want to talk about Lay Speaking call me. I would love for you to get involved in our schools." She had signed her name and her title "Miss. Conference Director Lay Speaking".

I almost fell off of my seat - then I smiled and thought, "that is just how God works. He placed that lady in the audience that day and then He urged me to speak out in front of all of those people and tell them about my desire to become a Lay Speaker. I never dreamed the "Director of Lay Speaking from the Miss. Conference" was in the audience listening to me. Thanks Mary, for being there that day and for taking the initiative to write me that little note that meant so much to me. As I keep saying - "God knows what He is doing". All we have to do is let him work in our lives and try to follow the direction in which He leads us.

Thank you again God......

My recovery from surgery went well. I think Dr. Billups and his nurse were surprised how well I got along. I healed well and was amazed the scarring was not worse. I had heard that some women have very bad scarring and some of them had sunk in places in their chest. I can say I was pleasingly surprised at the way my chest looked. Thanks to God I haven't even missed my breasts and that is unbelievable also. I will tell you women reading this that when you first dress and you can't wear a bra you will have to be a little creative in order to look normal.....

The doctor removed my staples and two drainage tubes in one week and the other drainage tubes the second week. I was glad to see those tubes go because they are so inconvenient. Now I knew that in three short weeks I would begin chemo therapy again. I would have to have four more chemos after surgery because I had lymph nodes involved. It would be a different type from the first round. It wouldn't be as strong, thank goodness, but it would have it's effects on my body in other ways.

I prayed about the upcoming chemo as I had prayed about everything else so far. I would put it in God's hands too.

CHAPTER XIV
"Second Round of Chemo Proves To Be A Breeze"

And so, after he had patiently endured, he obtained the promise.

Hebrews 6:15

By the time it was time to begin my second round of chemo I had recovered from the surgery really well, I had lost about seven pounds which I feel was fluid caused by the steroids they give you when they give you the chemo. I was really feeling pretty good for a change. The first four chemos were so strong and as they say "it not only kills the bad cells it kills your good cells as well", which really drags you down and makes you tired. But by now all that was out of my system and I felt pretty good. BUT, I would now begin a new type of chemo and have four rounds of it. I was ready to get started so that I could soon have this chemo behind me.

I met with Dr. Keady and he said we would have the four final rounds of chemo and it would be accompanied by a drip that is designed to hopefully keep the cancer from returning. Then once the chemo was completed I would have radiation to the left side of my chest. As I told you the right breast had been healed before surgery so I don't have to have radiation in that area.

The four chemos turned out to be a breeze. The only problem I experienced were with my legs which I had been warned about. I had a lot of swelling in my feet and legs and pain there as well; but I really don't want to complain because God has blessed me so much since I was diagnosed. I don't have a complaint compared to some people that have gone through chemo.

Pretty quickly my chemo was finally finished. I took my last chemo in May, 2006, Radiation would come next and I would still look to my God to carry me through as He had done so far.

I am standing on all of God's promises that I can find in my bible to get me completely through this journey. I know that God cannot lie and He will not break His promises. I have found God's promise Chapter 1, Verse 9 of Nahem which tells me that God will put an utter end - and that affliction WILL NOT rise up a second time. Therefore, I am trusting in this, God's promise, and I can be sure that this cancer will leave and stay in remission and never return to me at all.....

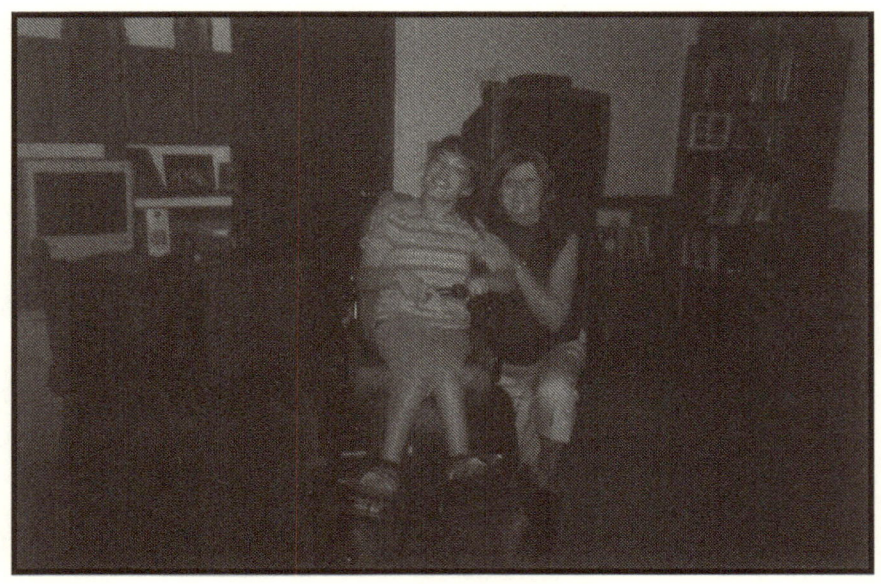

Chelsea and Cathy the day they sang to the Lord together.

CHAPTER XV
"My Special Friend And Cousin, Chelsea"

Oh come, let us sing unto the Lord; let us make

A joyful noise to the rock of our salvation.

(Psalm 95:1)

As I have told you I began singing for my Lord about one year prior to my being diagnosed with breast cancer. For that I am so thankful because singing makes me feel good, gives me strength and I feel closer to my Lord when I sing. My nephew sent me a card shortly after he found out that I was singing solos in church. The card had a verse written on it that said, "She who sings, prays twice"…I had never thought of singing in that respect but if you will give it some thought it is true. The songs have such a message in them and so many of the words are communication about and with our God..Now I love to sing and think about the fact that not only am I praising God in song but I am praying as well…

All through my illness I have tried to think of others and keep a prayer list beside me so that I can spend time praying for others. I think that is very important, especially when we, ourselves, are sick and in need of healing. I believe if we pray for others that God will gladly answer our prayers not only for those people but also for us as well.

My husband's cousin lives right across the road from us. Jackie has a granddaughter that has Cerebal Palsy but goes through life, with God's help, as if she has no disability at all. She enjoys school and loves get-togethers and parties with friends and family. She is a beautiful sixteen year old young lady named Chelsea. I have loved her so much since the first day I met her. She has the prettiest teeth and hair you have ever seen. She smiles all of the time and is a blessing not only to me but to everyone she meets.

I had been told that she was praying about my cancer and Jackie had told me that Chelsea loved to sing too. She had sung at her church also. I decided one day that I would call them and see if I could come over after school and spend some time with them and sing for Chelsea.

By this time I was over my mastectomy and was still taking chemo. It was my hope that I would somehow be a blessing to Chelsea that day by coming and singing for her.

Well, she let me sing for her and she sang for me and we even sang together. Little did I know when I went to see her to "bless her" that she would be such a blessing to me. She sang and it brought tears to my eyes because it touched my heart so much to watch her hold that microphone and sing for her Lord.

I was the one who received the blessing that day and I was the one whose spirits were lifted up…God did this for me..He used Chelsea, a child, to give me such a blessing that I needed that day. God knew I was trying to help someone and in turn that person helped me. That's how God works you know.

Just to see Chelsea smile and sing, knowing that when she was a young child they didn't even know if she would ever be able to talk, much less sing. God has blessed her and in turn she blesses others.

I appreciate Chelsea's love and support and will always cherish the memory of the day we sang to our Lord together. May God continue to bless my dear Chelsea and her family. And I thank you Lord for sending Chelsea our way.

CHAPTER XVI
"No Choice About Taking Radiation"

I had to wait a few weeks after my last chemo before meeting with the Radiation Doctor. My first appointment with Dr. Anderson came around pretty soon and he explained to me that some women have a choice as to whether to take radiation or not but "I didn't have a choice". There were several reasons by I didn't have a choice; the size of the primary tumor in my left breast, the fact that it was a stage 3 cancer and the fact that I had five of nine lymph nodes involved. Again I realized that I was in a life-threatening situation. He did tell me that people often ask him if he is going to burn them up and he said he was going to burn me up. He told me I would need 28 radiations and I would come to the clinic every day Monday through Friday. I thought to myself that this would probably seem like an eternity before it would be over. Dr. Anderson did tell me he was going to cure me and that if there were any cancer cells left in that surgical area that he wanted to kill them.

I would like to say that Dr. Anderson and all the other staff in the radiation clinic were wonderful. I never dreaded my treatments and actually enjoyed seeing and talking to all of them each day. I met other cancer patients as well and we shared our stories…Before I knew it I was at the end of the radiation treatments. I was weak during the time I was on treatments but I was accustomed to that with chemo. By the time I had completed the radiation, I was, in fact, burned up. I had a huge "scab" on my left side. The left side of my chest was red and it looked like it was very painful, but God did not allow me to hurt bad at all. The scab finally peeled away and left pretty pink new skin. He carried me through all of my treatments in such a remarkable way. Isn't He wonderful?

I was referred back to my cancer Dr. (Dr. Keady). He told me that he was going to give me a drip once a month for 6 months and that I would take the cancer drug Tamoxifen for five years in hopes that the cancer will not return. My lab work and chest x-rays are showing that the cancer has not spread to my liver, bones or lungs. I feel great. God has healed me from this breast cancer.

My surgery report tells me that I have a stage three invasive ductal carcinoma and that I have five of nine metastatic lymph nodes involved. I do not have early detected breast cancer. Everything I read that pertains to breast cancer says that you have a better chance of survival if your cancer is early detected breast cancer, which mine is not. All medical reports indicate that it almost always spreads or metastasizes. BUT, everything I read in my bible tells me all of God's promises and that He wants me healed and He wants me to have a long, abundant life. So I am standing on my God's promises that "by His stripes I am healed". I am healed as of the writing of this book. God answered our prayers for my healing... I am believing Him that He will keep me well and that the cancer will never return or spread anywhere in me.

I did follow through and go to Lay Speaking School in September, 2006 because I feel that God has called me to do that. I have made up may mind that I will not die an early death but live and declare the works of my Lord.........

The real purpose of this book not only is to tell you just how awesome God is and just how very much He has blessed me through my breast cancer journey - but it is also written to hopefully be a help to each of you reading it. I want to let you know that wherever you go, whatever you do, whatever trial comes your way God will carry you through it.

CHAPTER XVII

My Friend, Mary, Loses Her Battle With Breast Cancer

"There is no man that hath power over the spirit to retain the spirit; neither hath he power in the day of death.

(Ecclesiastes 8:7)

I had worked with a lady named Mary while I was employed at East Miss. State Hospital all those years. After I was diagnosed with breast cancer I had talked to Mary about her breast cancer. She had been diagnosed about eight months prior to me receiving my diagnosis. I'll never forget the words she spoke to me the first time we talked after my diagnosis. She said, "Cathy we have worked too hard to just lay down and die".

She did great for two years and then a mutual friend told me that Mary had been real sick for a couple of weeks. Once Mary got back to work I called her and she told me that she had gall bladder problems, nothing cancer related. I was so happy it wasn't the cancer again because I knew, like me, she had lymph node involvement and the cancer could reoccur.

After talking to her, about a week later she was hospitalized and they found that the cancer had, in fact, returned to her liver. My heart was broken, not only for Mary, but for me, because I thought if Mary lived I would live and if she died I would die. The devil filled me with fear immediately. He said "Mary isn't going to make it and you won't either." Now you know I had been fighting the devil during this whole journey, and now he was back again.

All I could think about was Mary and her family. I received e-mails from a friend that kept me posted on how Mary was doing because I knew I didn't need to call her, she was so sick. I did send her cards to let her know we were praying for her total recovery. I prayed so very hard for Mary. I prayed day and night that she would survive.

Then I received the news that she was at home and not expected to live. I received a call early one morning that Mary had gone to be with her Lord. I was so sad because I knew how bad Mary wanted to live to see her son graduate next year.

I didn't understand why God didn't answer my prayers for her total recovery. I cried a lot. Then I snapped back and began thinking that God did give Mary two good years after the diagnosis and I know the bible says we all have a time to be born and a time to die. That is completely out of our control.

I renewed my strength and my faith in my God and I have decided that for Mary and what she said to me that day I will fight even harder to live and beat this breast cancer. I know in my heart that Mary is at peace now and has been reunited with family that had gone on before her. I know she was happy to sit at the feet of Jesus also. I love Mary and I appreciate her encouraging words that she spoke to me after my diagnosis. She gave me so much hope through my chemo, surgery and radiation. I know God will bless her in a special way for doing that for me.

As I've told you before, God knows what is best for us and he guides us and orchestrates our lives. As it turned out Mary died on a Monday night and visitation at the funeral home was going to be Wednesday night. My daughter was scheduled to go out of town on business and she needed me to come a day earlier to Florida to take care of Cody. I always go every other Thursday but it was necessary for me to go on Wednesday this particular week. I was upset that I wasn't going to get to go to the funeral home or the funeral. Then a nurse friend of mine, Linda, wrote me an e-mail and told me that "God orchestrates our lives and that He knew I didn't need to be around death but that I needed to be around the living; and who better to spur me on than Cody."

I knew she was right and that I especially didn't need to attend a funeral of someone that had breast cancer like me. I told several friends what she had said and they totally agreed. This was not the first time that God orchestrated my life and I'm very sure it won't be the last.

The purpose of this chapter is to tell you that God does not always answer our prayers the way we ask them but God does answer in a way that He feels is the best for us. I have seen that many times in my life. Mary had just turned 48 years old and that seems so young to die, but I do believe God knows what's best for us and we just have to trust Him in everything.

I will continue to pray that cancer can someday be snuffed completely out and no one will ever have to go through this mean illness again.

I do thank God that once we found out Mary was dieing we began to pray that He would be merciful and take her painlessly and peacefully. I was told that the prayers were answered and she went peacefully at the end. Thank you God for that answered prayer. Please, to everyone reading this, never give up. Keep your eyes on Jesus. Even though there are those falling around you it is important that you keep your eyes on Jesus so that He can carry you through miraculously. He can and He will.

I continue to read my bible, pray and focus on my Lord. I continue to have treatments each week to try to keep the cancer from returning. The treatments will be over in April, 2007. Some people have continued to take these drips until the cancer returned but it is so dangerous for the heart that my doctor feels it is not in my best interest to do that. I trust my cancer Dr. He is very smart and I also trust my Lord to take care of me even after the drips are discontinued.

The rest of this book will be devoted to bible verses, inspirational statements, etc. that somehow will help you, guide and direct you in the paths you should take to help you have a closer walk with your best friend and your master and the biggest source of help you will EVER have or EVER need when you are wallowing in the lowest points of your life.

CHAPTER XVIII
Meditating On God's Word Will Help You

Now that I have told you my personal story about my journey through breast cancer, I want to tell you that it is absolutely amazing that we have such an Awesome God.

I want everyone who is reading this book to be reassured and reminded that no matter what trial comes into your life, that you will make it because of the love and help of our God.

Please get into your bible and study and find God's promises. There are promises from God all through our bible not only pertaining to healing but also regarding many things in our lives such as finances, marriage, etc. When we are at the lowest point of our lives we may feel that we have no strength to pray. That was true for me during chemo. This is a time that we can depend on friends and family to pray for us. We can depend on other people's prayers to get us through.

Once you have regained your strength though, you need to begin your communication with God through prayer and meditation. When you pray you have to have faith and believe that God will hear and answer your prayers. Prayer without faith will do you no good. Believe in God for what you need and you will have it.

The bible says that "if two of you agree on earth concerning anything that they ask, it will be done for them by my Father in Heaven. (Matthew 18:19)

I know that many people have agreed for my healing and staying healed, so I have faith in God that it will be done for me.

Remember that the devil will be there taunting you and trying to beat your faith in God down. You will have to resist the devil. Always rebuke the devil and tell him you have someone much stronger on your side and you are living for God no matter what happens.

During this journey through cancer I have had pain, weakness, depression, stress, etc., and I had to rebuke the devil and keep my eyes on Jesus to see me through it; and He has and will continue to. I read a statement just the other day that said "if God brings you to it, He will get you through it", and that is so true.

I am not a strong person. I take that back; I didn't think I was a strong person until this journey. God has made me strong and able to cope with every bit of "this hand I have been dealt in my life".

If I had not known about God, the bible and how important they are, I would have never made it this far. If you are struggling with an illness, please never give up. God wants to heal you and make you well and He wants to bless you with a long, abundant life whereby you can declare the works of the Lord. (Psalm 118:17)

I prayed and asked God to keep His promise to give me a long abundant life. I reminded Him that I need to live to witness for Him and declare His works to others and that I cannot witness from the grave. I am sure He heard me, as He always does, and that He will honor that request.

Everything I read about cancer and other illnesses tells me that we do not need stress in our lives if we want to be well and/or healed. We must de-stress our lives. One way to do that is to find things that make us happy or make us laugh. Laughter is as good as medicine. It has it's healing affects. Try everything that you can to help you be positive and happy in your life. Laugh often and even laugh to the point you lose your breath. I have started renting comedy movies and reading the funny's in the newspaper. It is also good to think of things in your life, for instance when you were growing up, etc, that made you happy or made you laugh. These happy thoughts and memories will relieve pressure and have a calming affect which will be a positive thing for you.

I know that in the book I read by Dodie Osteen and her survival from liver cancer, she said that it was very important that we pray for others as well as for ourselves. She reminded me that James 5:16 says "pray for one another that you may be healed". I do keep a prayer list and pray for others daily and find that I really enjoy doing that and I feel a great satisfaction from doing that. It also is great to know that I will receive my healing because I care for others and pray for others. I notice I always feel better after praying for others and I have seen my prayers for others answered and that is an absolutely wonderful feeling.

We know that we must pray and believe that God will answer. Everyone that knows me hears me say I have "perfect faith" because as far as I am concerned "it is as good as done" when I ask in faith. This doesn't mean that I always feel confident and never worry. It is human nature, unfortunately, to worry; but God does not want us to worry. He wants us to wait on Him to answer in His time. His time is not the same as our time. We tend to want our answer pronto, right now, immediately...God makes us wait to teach us patience.

God's lessons are not always easy. As a matter of fact, most of them are very hard; but that is part of growing up in Christ. Just as we were children growing up and learning lessons from our earthly father, we must grow spiritually through lessons from our Heavenly Father.

Life is God's greatest gift to us. We need to move through the days of our lives reading and meditating on God's word. Even driving in our cars or sitting in line somewhere we can turn our thoughts to God, our friend.

Scriptures that helped me through this journey of breast cancer and that I believe will help you also, no matter what you problem is, are the following: (These are taken from my Living Bible)

What is faith? It is the confident assurance that something we want is going to happen. It is the certainty that what we hope for is waiting for us, even though we cannot see it up ahead.

Hebrews 11:1:

Oh Lord, my God, I pleaded with you and you gave me my health again. You brought me back from the brink of the grave, from death itself, and here I am alive!

Psalms 30:2 - 3:

He spoke, and they were healed - snatched from the door of death.

Psalms 107:20:

But He was wounded and bruised for our sins. He was chastised that we might have peace, He was lashed - and we were healed.

Isaiah 53:5:

Lord, you alone can heal me, you alone can save and my praises are for you alone.

Jeremiah 17:14:

He personally carried the load of our sins in His own body when He died on the cross, so that we can be finished with sin and live a good life from now on. For His wounds have healed ours!

I Peter 2:24:

I also tell you this – if two of your agree down here on earth concerning anything you ask for, my Father in Heaven wil do it for you.

Matthew 18:19:

I will satisfy him with a full life and give him my salvation.

Psalm 91:16:

I have set before you life or death, blessing or curse. Oh, that you would choose life; that you and your children might live! Choose to love the Lord your God and to obey Him and to cling to Him, for He is your life and the length of your days.

Deuteronomy 30:19 - 20:

Look, a leper is approaching. He kneels before Him, worshipping "Sir", the leper pleads, "if you want to, you can heal me". Jesus touches the man, "I want to", He says, "Be healed", and instantly the leprosy disappears.

Matthew 8:2 - 3:(It is God's will for you to be healed)

Listen, son of mine, to what I say, listen carefully. Keep these thoughts ever in mind; let them penetrate deep within your heart for they will mean real life for you and radiant health.

Proverbs 4:20 - 22:

Since I have had cancer and been singing and witnessing for God, my mothers pastor told me and the congregation that He has prayed and asked God to reward me for my faith. He also asked the congregation to pray that same prayer for me. I appreciate those prayers. Hebrews 10:35 says, "Do not throw away your confidence, it will be richly rewarded".

It is during our trials that we learn to depend on God. He wants us to lean on Him always. His grace is sufficient for us!

The thief (satan) comes only to steal our joy and take our life. We cannot let Him. Our God is more powerful than satan so rebuke satan, lean on God and live expecting your miracle from Him.

We need to thank God for every day we have. He makes our days and is our hope for each new day.

My prayer is that this, my first book, has in some way helped you or encouraged you as you face problems in your life. I am living proof that if we trust the Lord we can be confident that in His time He will turn things around for us. We need to "rest in the Lord" and while we wait on Him we must stay busy studying His word, praying, praising Him, and staying in conscious union with our Lord and Savior, Jesus Christ. You are never alone. He is as near as your next breath.

I am believing God for my permanent healing of this breast cancer. As of Now, March, 2007, all of my tests show that I am cancer free. I know that we all have a time to be born and a time to die.

I want everyone reading this book to know it is important that we live our lives in such a way that we will be prepared to die when our time comes, with the assurance that we will go to Heaven to be with God.

I am living my life praising God at all times and in all things. I will continue singing for God at every opportunity as well as witnessing for Him. I tell God now, "Not my will but Thine be done". I am confident that God knows what is best for us and as our loving Father, He will do what is best for us always!

To my family and friends I want you to know that when the Lord chooses to call me home, I am confident that I will be sheltered in the arms of God because "it is well with my soul".....God bless you all

With all my love, *Cathy*

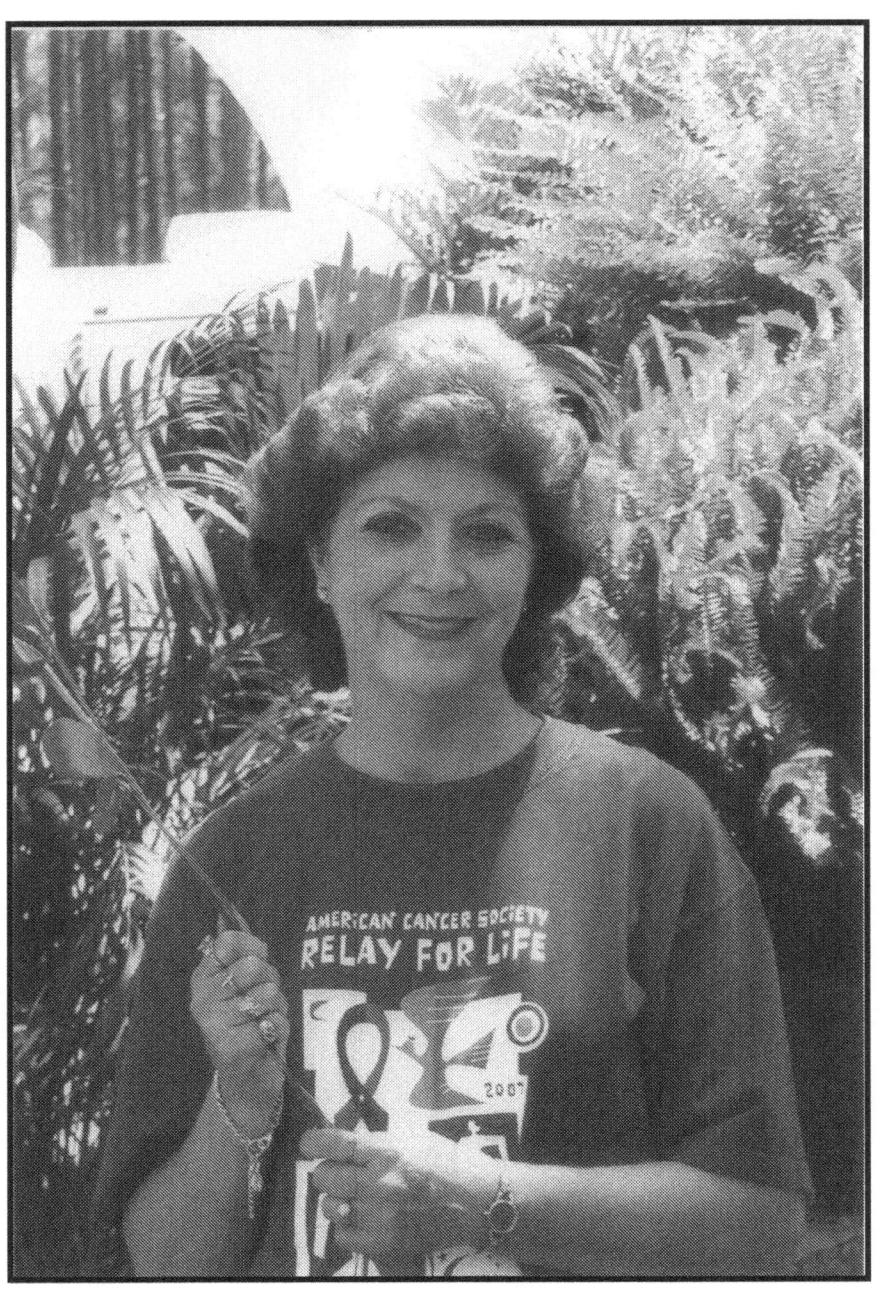

Cathy at Clarke Co. Relay for Life where she sang.

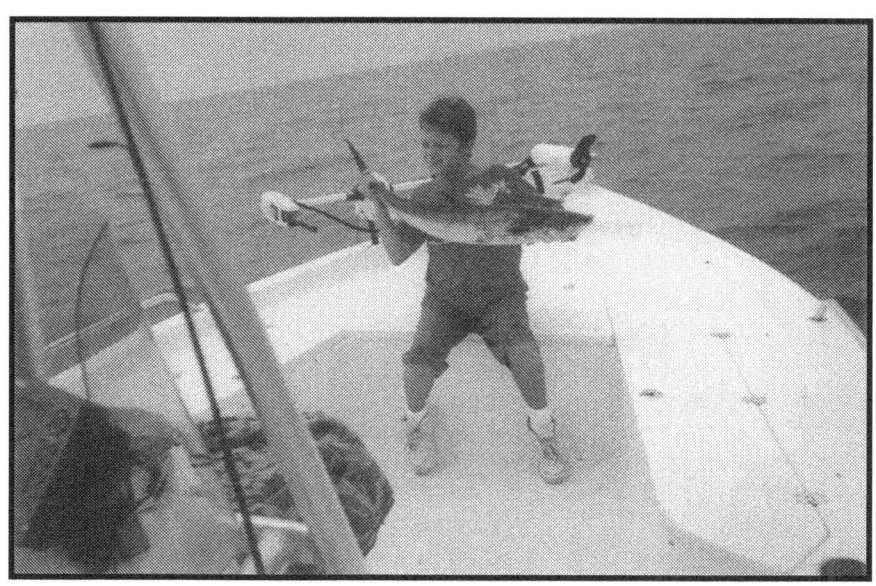

Cathy's grandson, Cody, on a deep sea fishing trip his mom gave him for his 11th birthday. Those who went with him that day were: his mom, Karen, memaw Cathy and papaw Randy. FUN…

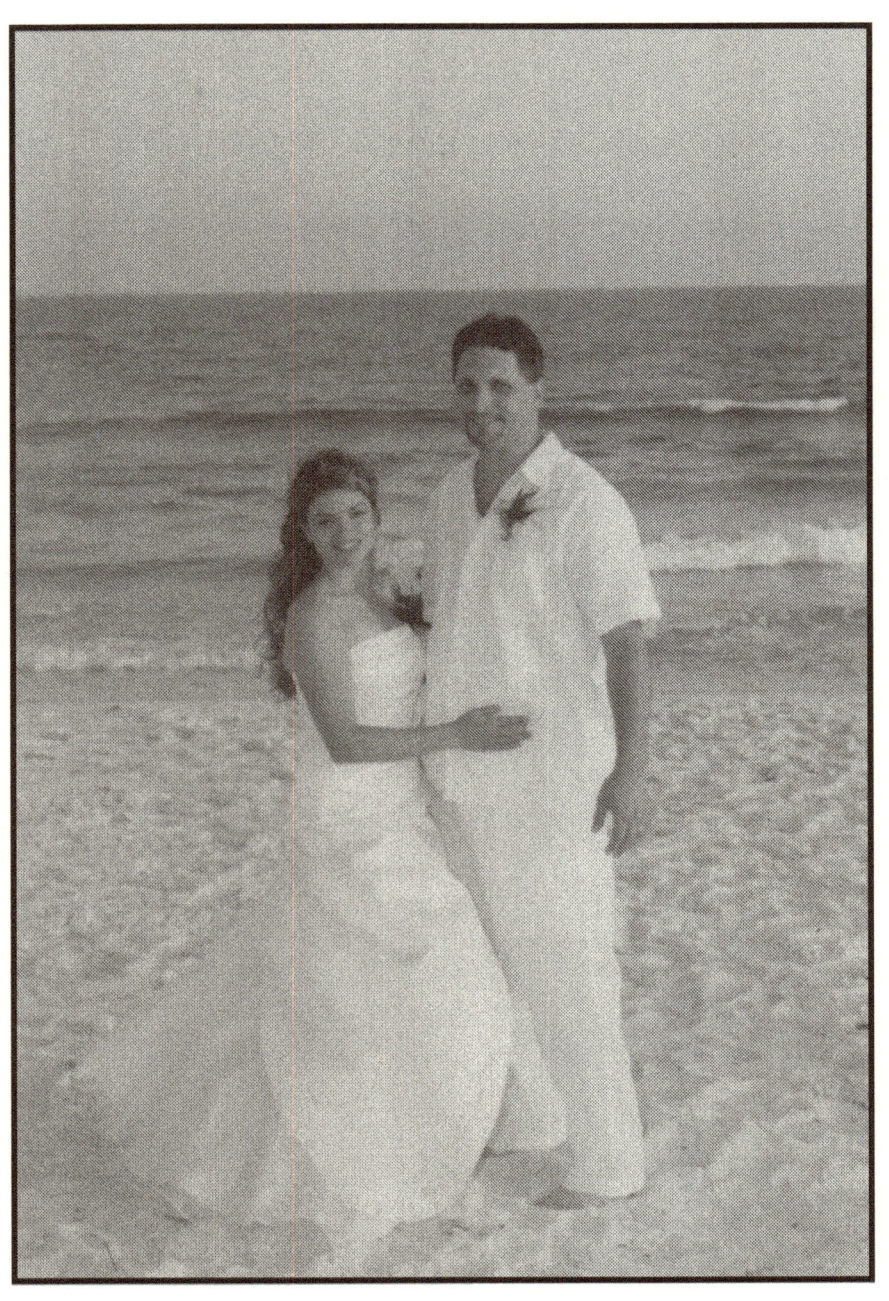

Karen and John at their beach wedding May 5, 2007. Cathy was well and able to attend that day.

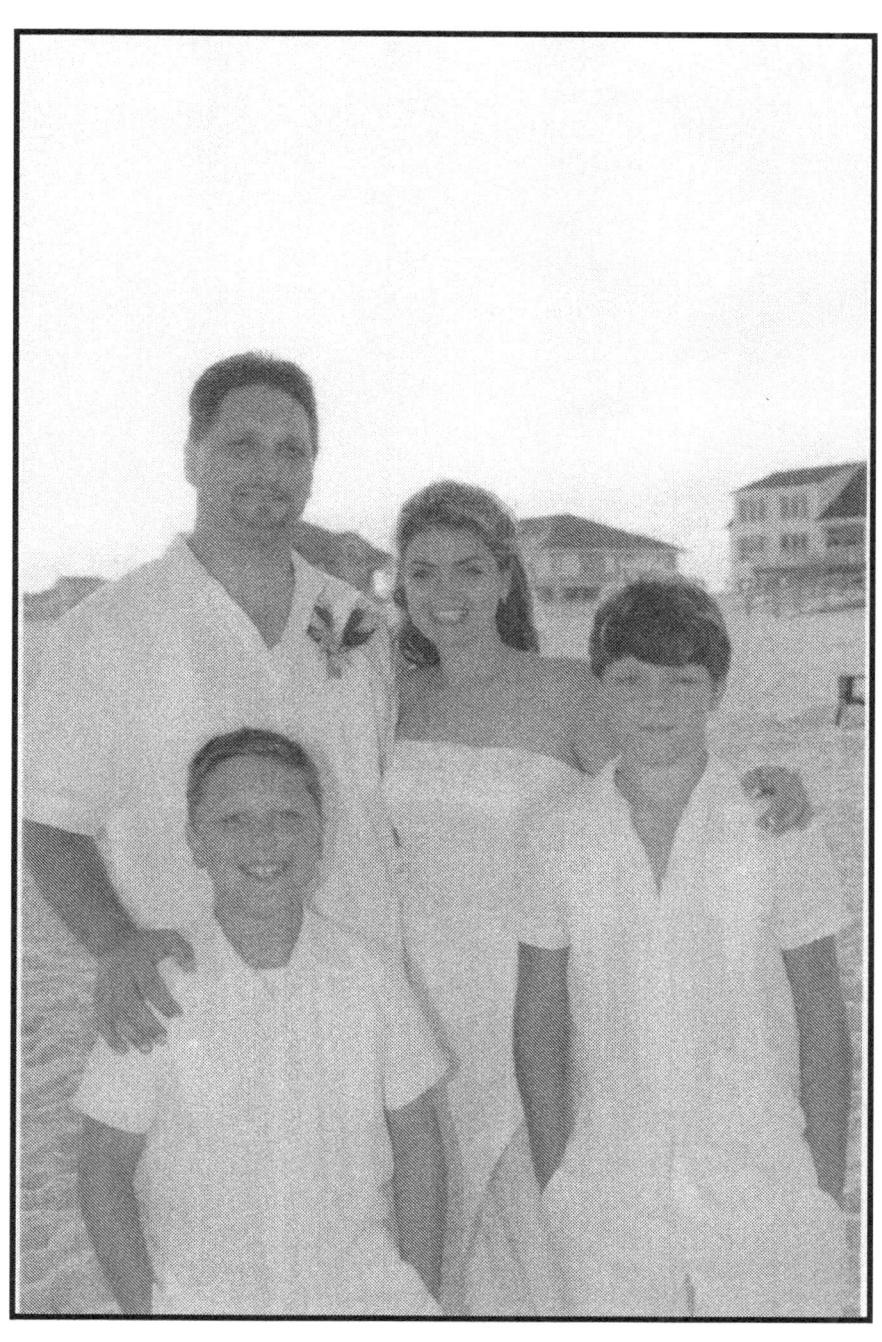

John and Karen at their beach wedding with John's son, Brian (left) and Karen's son, Cody (right).

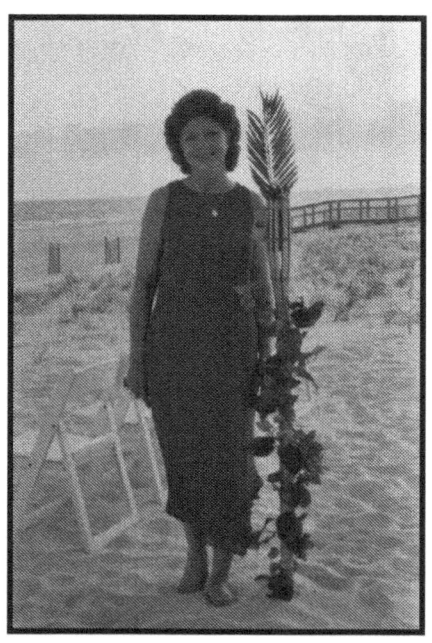

CATHY SUITOR RILEY is a 56 year old woman who was diagnosed with bi-lateral invasive and non-invasive ductal carcinoma when she was 54 years old. The day she was diagnosed it was found that she had several tumors in both breasts and in her lymph nodes and she felt like her life would end very, very soon...

Cathy is a woman of strong faith and her faith has grown even more during this breast cancer journey. This is her first book but she plans to write more books in the future. Cathy is very aware that her type of diagnosis does not hold a very good prognosis according to all medical statistics, but she also knows that Her God is the same yesterday, today and always. God healed in bible days and He can do the same today.

This author is praying that God will heal her and keep her healed from cancer so that she can declare the works of the Lord. She is working for the Lord by singing and witnessing for Him every chance she gets. Cathy cannot get enough of telling others how good God has been to her all of her life, especially during this journey. It was so obvious that God sent friends, family and even strangers at exactly the right time to deliver messages of hope from God. The pastors and congregations of Coopers Chapel Methodist Church, Hawkins Memorial Methodist Church, Wesley Chapel Methodist Church and Christian Fellowship Church were faithful encouragers to Cathy during her illness, treatments and surgery. She knows they were all "God Sent"....

She has a grown daughter, Karen, and a grandson, Cody, that give her the will to live and with God's help she will live a long and healthy life.